Praise for

"Would you like your life to be both healthier and happier? Dina Colman's guidance will get you there. Her voice is clear, wise and reliable. Heed it and you'll be on your way to true wellness."

— **JOHN ROBBINS**
author of *Diet For A New America*,
co-founder of the Food Revolution Network,
FoodRevolution.org

"*Four Quadrant Living* is a simple, clear introduction to an Integral lifestyle, with recommendations covering all four quadrants (psychospiritual, behavioral, communal, and systemic). These basic dimensions are present in all humans, and are there whether we know it or not, want it or not—and we can treat them in ways that lead to health, or ways that lead to illness. Dina Colman includes practices and exercises (and advice in general) that will help insure the result is health, not illness, and a life filled with more joy, vitality, strength, wellness, and happiness. If you're looking for a way to improve your life, this is a terrific place to begin."

— **KEN WILBER**
author of *The Integral Vision*

"Dina Colman's *Four Quadrant Living* is as close to being an 'owners manual' for being a mindful human being as I've ever seen. Living a holistic life in this day and age is not just a good idea, it's a prerequisite if you want to live a healthy, balanced life. We all have the choice to live a higher quality of life than we do, and this book serves as a great check list for how to create that level of life experience we all crave. Dina is precise and practical in her explanations and suggestions. *Four Quadrant Living* is nothing short of a great 'reset' button to keep your everyday life on track and moving in the direction of high quality living. If everyone lived the way Dina suggests, none of us would recognize the planet we currently live on. For me, it would be a dream come true."

— **DANNY DREYER**
author of *Chi Running, Chi Walking,* and *Chi Marathon,*
founder of Chi Living

"Once in a while a book comes along that helps a generation of readers access a new way of living—not by implementing major changes, but by making minor tweaks that change everything. This is such a book. In the most accessible and inviting language, Dina Colman has assembled a small book of simple but profound wisdom, complete with the suggestions needed to bring about change. Whether you are just starting out on the journey to simplify your life and find more meaning, or you are deeply involved in a spiritual practice, this book offers tools for everyday living that all of us need to be reminded of now and then. It's a book that feels like a conversation with a close friend from the moment you open it, and is one that many readers will keep by their bedside for years to come. I know a few dozen people I'd like to give this to, and I bet you will too."

— **SARAH SUSANKA**
author of *The Not So Big House* series and *The Not So Big Life*

"Dina Colman provides the top-level strategy to do the right things the right way to change your life."

— GUY KAWASAKI
author of *APE: Author, Publisher, Entrepreneur*,
former chief evangelist of Apple

"*Four Quadrant Living* is a guide for taking charge of the style in which we live our lives. It is about lifestyle medicine. As Dina Colman wisely points out, contrary to common belief, our genes only rarely determine our destiny. However, what we think, how we live our lives, the relationships we nurture, and the environment we live in, all have surprisingly powerful effects on our health. This practical, easy-to-read book is a must read if you want to take charge of your health."

— LEN SAPUTO
author of *A Return to Healing*,
DoctorSaputo.com

"For millennia, sages, mystics and wisdom keepers have reminded us of the importance of the four quadrants of life. In today's world of countless distractions and cyber cacophony, Dina's book, *Four Quadrant Living*, is a wonderful and refreshing synthesis of great wisdom, fruitful experience and good common sense which we would all do well to follow."

— BRIAN LUKE SEAWARD, Ph.D.
author of *Managing Stress* and *Stand Like Mountain, Flow Like Water*

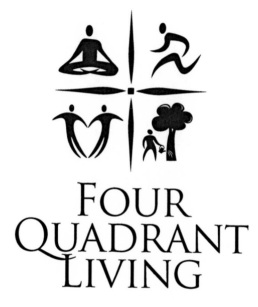

FOUR QUADRANT LIVING

Dear Christy,
Thank you for your support.
It has been fun to get to
know you. Wishing you
abundant health + happiness!
Dina

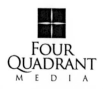

FOUR QUADRANT LIVING

Making Healthy Living
Your New Way of Life

Dina Colman

Dina Colman
10/12/13

FOUR
QUADRANT
M E D I A

Published by Four Quadrant Media
An Imprint of Wyatt-MacKenzie

ISBN: 9781939288226
Library of Congress Control Number: 2013944717

Printed in the United States of America

For my sister, Debbie

*The grace and strength you showed during your illness
will always be an inspiration to me. I am grateful every day
that you are healthy and in my life.*

TABLE OF CONTENTS

Mind.
PART ONE

Body.
PART TWO

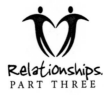

Relationships.
PART THREE

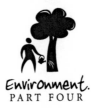

Environment.
PART FOUR

APPENDIX

FOREWORD

I volunteered to write this foreword. I don't know the author, and we have never met. But I liked this book. A lot. And I want to tell you why.

Sometimes we feel damaged and limited. By genetics, fate, or fortune. We may feel life has loaded the dice against us. Our measuring rod is our health. It is sometimes a cause to lament. *"My health is much worse, this year."* It is sometimes a consolation. *"Well, at least you've got your health."*

Health is, above all, an experience. That's how we talk about it. *"I've experienced good health."* Or *"I've experienced remarkable healing."* Dina, our author here, has had that experience dramatically, over a number of years, and now, turning outward, thinking of others, she has decided not to keep this to herself. She has pressed into service here, her own experience, her sister's and her clients' experiences as well, plus quotations, research, statistics, step-by-step instructions, common sense, and pep-talks, to help you experience what she has.

And her prescription? Well, it isn't just three points you need to keep in mind. Or five. Or even ten. If you made a list of everything she includes in her prescription here, you'd have just about everything but the kitchen sink. She covers so much ground. Even in this short book.

Far from being intimidated by her long list, this is exactly why I like this book. This is not just a book about how to improve your health. I wouldn't trust it, if it was. This is a book about how to do Life. Those two—health and life—are inseparable. Anyone who writes about health, and doesn't realize that, still has a lot to learn.

I am 86 (so far). There are days when health seems to me to be just a symptom. Or a barometer, if you will. Of life.

You can't always control your health. But you can improve it. And how do you do that? By improving the way you do Life. Her experience, her prescription? There are four quadrants to life that you need to pay particular attention to.

She has learned you need to pay attention to—and work on—all four. Not just three of them, nor two, nor one. All four. Pay more attention to—and work on—what's going on in your Mind. Pay more attention to—and work on—what's going on in your Body. Pay more attention to—and work on—what's going on in your Relationships. Pay more attention to—and work on—what's going on in your Surroundings (i.e. Environment). She'll show you how.

Deal with all four the best you can, laugh a lot, sleep a lot, love a lot, and your resulting improvement in health will be your testament and your barometer of how well you're doing Life—the best life, under the circumstances, the most victorious life.

I got some great ideas, from this book. I need them. After all, I may still have a long way to go.

Dick Bolles
Author, *What Color Is Your Parachute? A Practical Manual for Job-Hunters & Career-Changers*

∾

PREFACE

Fifteen years ago, when I was 30, doctors told me that I had an 87% chance of getting breast cancer in my lifetime. I was told this as my sister, Debbie, made her way through chemotherapy, stem cell transplant, surgery, and radiation. At age 32, Debbie had been diagnosed with stage 3 breast cancer. These events changed my life.

Prior to this time, I was climbing the corporate ladder. I had earned a master's degree in business administration, and I was working as a marketing manager at Hewlett Packard. Life was good. I had no knowledge or concern about healthy living. My relationship with health changed the day I received the phone call from Debbie.

As I watched my sister go through the debilitating treatment, I was overcome by fear—fear that my sister would die and that cancer would be my fate as well. Because my sister was so young and her cancer was so aggressive, doctors wondered if the disease ran in our family. It turns out, it did. Nine relatives within the last three generations were identified as having breast cancer at some point in their lives.

When I learned that I am at high risk for cancer, I worried about every morsel of food that went into my body and every product that touched my skin. Although I began eating healthy foods and using healthy products, I was not healthy because I was operating out of fear. I was developing an unhealthy obsession with healthy living. My fear of disease and dying were overpowering my joy in living.

After recovering from a year of treatment, Debbie started to look and feel like herself again. With time, the intense fear I had felt subsided. Still, the statistics quoted to me about my possible fate floated in and out of my consciousness as the years passed. Was cancer my destiny, or did I have a say in the matter? This nagging question eventually changed the direction of my life. A decade after finding out about my genetically based high risk, I left the corporate world and went back to school to find the answer.

Earning my master's degree in holistic health education taught me that how I live my life *does* impact my health. It *is* possible to create a new health destiny! Eating well, exercising often, thinking positively, having fun, managing stress, being in nurturing relationships, and living in a clean environment are all health-supporting actions that counterbalance our genetics.

Fifteen years later, my sister is cancer-free and I continue to beat the odds. I no longer live in fear. Instead, I've chosen empowerment. You can do it, too.

Inspired by my new knowledge, I founded my company, Four Quadrant Living, to help others live healthier and happier lives. The four quadrants of healthy living are Mind, Body, Relationships, and Environment. For true health and wellness, we need to nurture all four quadrants, not just one.

Living well doesn't only apply to reducing the risk of breast cancer, it also applies to many other health concerns like diabetes, high blood pressure, heart disease, allergies, autoimmune disorders, and more. Studies show that many of these chronic diseases *are* preventable.

It can be overwhelming with all of the noise and confusion out there about how to live healthy. So many of the "solutions" are short-term fixes that aren't sustainable or enjoyable. I've tried in this book to sort through it all and get down to the basics—to provide you with tools, tips, and ideas for making healthy living a way of life.

One big lesson I've learned is that an important part of health is pleasure. Healthy living that isn't fun defeats the purpose and won't last. Remember to have fun in the process of trying out some of the ideas in this book.

In the chapters that follow, you will find simple, effective, and natural ways to take control of your health so that you feel empowered, beat the odds, and live radiantly.

Dina Colman, MA, MBA
Danville, CA
October 2013

~

INTRODUCTION

I grew up with two "truths" that I now realize simply aren't true.

First, I believed that health is all about the physical. Mainstream American medicine addresses only one quadrant—the body. Our physical illnesses are believed to spring from physical causes and are treated with physical interventions, such as surgery and medication. Recently, behavior modifications like diet and exercise have been included as well. We take medications to mask the symptoms, but too often we don't get to the root of the problem.

This is a limiting view of health. Health is a state that emerges from four areas—four quadrants—Mind, Body, Relationships, and Environment. We may be eating well and exercising, but we cannot truly be healthy if at the same time our mind is stressed, our relationships are toxic, and our world is sick.

Second, I believed that our genes are our destiny. My dad often used the phrase, "It's in my genes" whenever he talked about his heart disease. After all, his father died of heart disease, as did six of his aunts and uncles. Whenever I asked him why he didn't exercise more or eat better, he would say that it didn't matter because his heart condition was genetic. Hearing this made me feel hopeless for him and for me. After all, if it was in *his* genes, it was in *mine* too.

Now all these years later, I've found out it's not true. Our genes are not our destiny; it is the combination of our genetics and environment that determines our health. It may not be the inherited genes that are causing the disease, but rather the inherited bad habits. How we live our life affects how our genes express themselves. Genes can be turned on and off by such influencers as injury, stress, diet, hormones, emotions, toxins, and infections. This activation of genes is called gene expression and has profound influence on health and disease.

These two ideas together are the genesis of this book and my company, Four Quadrant Living. For more information on the foundation of and inspiration for Four Quadrant Living, see *A Nod to Integral Theory and Epigenetics* at the end of this book.

~

In this country, our health practices are failing. Fifty percent of Americans have at least one chronic condition, such as cardio-vascular disease, cancer, diabetes, or obesity. Cancer hits almost one of every two people in the U.S., more than one-third of adults have prediabetes, and more than one-third of adults are obese. We spend close to three trillion dollars on health care in this country each year, 75% of which go toward these chronic illnesses.[1]

There is mounting research showing that our changes in diet and lifestyle over the past few decades have been contributing to these alarming statistics. We now eat more processed foods and trans fats, we are more sedentary, we are highly stressed, and we have more toxins in our environment.

Many scientists, nutritionists, doctors, and researchers have explored the connection between health and how we live. Here are a few highlights:

- As early as the 1930s, Dr. Weston Price, a dentist and nutri-tion pioneer, discovered that when native cultures adopted similar eating habits to those of more advanced societies, they began to suffer the same health problems of the modern world.

- In the 1950s, Roger Williams, Ph.D., coined the term "biochemical individuality," to represent the idea that each individual has distinct nutritional needs for optimal functioning. He pointed out that identical twins with the same DNA can have different gene expression, depending on external influences. He believed that it was the interaction between heredity and nutrition that determines our health.

- Jeffrey Bland, Ph.D., a leader in functional medicine, talks about genetic nutritioneering—the idea that how we live and what we eat can influence how our genes express themselves.

- Dr. Dean Ornish, a physician, has been directing clinical research for over 30 years, demonstrating that diet and lifestyle changes can prevent, and even reverse, heart disease. His preventative program has proven so effective that dozens of insurance companies now cover the cost of participation for their insureds.

- Bruce Lipton, Ph.D., a stem cell biologist, focuses his efforts on the influence of our subconscious thoughts on our health.

- John Robbins in *Healthy at 100* and Dan Buettner in *The Blue Zones* look at some of the healthiest and longest living people in the world and discover that it is their way of life, not their genetics, that is the secret to their success.

It is time to hold ourselves accountable for our health and take action by making changes to our dietary and lifestyle habits. Diseases like heart disease and cancer are in many cases preventable. It is estimated that over 30% of cancer and 80% of heart disease, stroke, and type 2 diabetes can be prevented.[2]

We have come to rely on the medical system instead of taking personal responsibility for our health. We are quick to go to the doctor or rely on medication at the slightest hint of feeling sick. The average American takes 12 prescription drugs annually. Over 10% of Americans aged 12 and older take anti-depressant medication. For women aged 40 to 60, it is almost one in four. Fewer than a quarter of those given the medication have been diagnosed with depression or anxiety disorders.[3] Most get the drug for what once were considered ordinary problems such as sleeping issues, moodiness, and relationship conflicts. We are medicating for things that can be healed naturally.

American mainstream medicine focuses on disease care, not health care, treating the symptoms rather than understanding and treating the underlying cause. For acute and trauma care, the tools and knowledge of traditional medicine are indispensable. However, for chronic illnesses, the current approach is not working optimally. If we spend more time promoting our health through living well, we will spend less time fighting disease with interventions such as drugs and surgery that can have harmful side effects. While doctors are taught about prescription drugs in medical school, they are educated very little about the impact that stress, nutrition, sleep, exercise, relationships, and environment have on our health.

We can learn by listening to the wise words of our ancestors. Voltaire, a French scholar in the 18th century, said, *"The art of medicine consists of keeping the patient amused while nature heals the disease."* Maimonides, a Jewish medical philosopher in the 12th century, said, *"Let nothing which can be treated by diet be treated by other means."* Hippocrates, an ancient Greek physician in 400 BC, is famously quoted as saying, *"Let food be thy medicine and medicine be thy food."* For thousands of years, we have known the power of healthy living.

∼

Living healthy doesn't need to be complicated. *Four Quadrant Living* provides simple and natural ways to live a healthy and happy life. The tools and tips provided will help you reduce stress, laugh more, live authentically, have more energy, take fewer medications, sleep better, have healthier relationships, reduce toxins, and more. The book consists of four parts, covering each of the four quadrants—Mind, Body, Relationships, and Environment. Within each part, there are 12 chapters. At the end of each section, there is a set of questions to help you identify which quadrants may need attention.

Part One, Mind, provides you with ideas for calming your mind. It includes techniques such as being mindful, breathing, thinking positively, and laughing, all of which reduce stress. This is essential for your health considering that the majority of doctor visits are for stress-related complaints.

Part Two, Body, suggests ways to nourish your body by feeding it well, giving it enough sleep, and using natural products. Numerous studies show the impact that nutrition, exercise, sleep, and other body factors have on our health.

Part Three, Relationships, offers you tips for removing the toxic relationships from your life and strengthening the supportive ones. Studies show that people with a strong social support network live longer and are healthier than those without.

Part Four, Environment, presents you with suggestions for detoxifying your environment and finding health in nature. Our health is intimately connected to the health of the environment. Toxins in the environment have been linked to numerous diseases and health conditions.

You can choose to read the chapters in order, or you can go straight to the quadrant you feel needs the most nourishment. Not all of the ideas will resonate with you. Focus on the ones that do, and set aside the rest for now. After you have mastered a few ideas, you can always go back through the book and try a few more. This process is about meeting yourself where you are at and making a few changes at a time, so that healthy living becomes a part of who you are, not just something you do.

This book is beneficial for you whether you currently have an illness or want to prevent one. If you have an illness, this book provides you with ideas for minimizing pain, conquering fear, taking back control, and nurturing your health in areas you may not have considered. If you are concerned about your health because a disease "runs in the family," this book will empower you so that you no longer feel resigned to your family's health history. If you do not currently have a health concern, this book provides you with ways to have a whole new relationship with health. You will experience greater energy and vitality, *and* you will be doing what you can to prevent health issues from arising. As Benjamin Franklin said, *"An ounce of prevention is worth a pound of cure."*

You have the power to promote health in your life—to create a new health destiny. Every day you make choices that impact your health when you select the foods you eat, the products you use, the exercise you do or don't do, the stress you allow, the people you surround yourself with, and the environment you live in. We may not have total control over our health, but we have enough to make a significant difference. Start Four Quadrant Living today to make healthy living your new way of life!

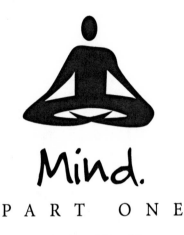

Mind.

PART ONE

Mind and Health

*O*ne evening, Marie went out for a run, as she did regularly. *Midway through the run, she intuitively felt that something wasn't right. She saw a man walking toward her, and even though he moved into the street to give her space, he made her nervous. His steps seemed calculated. She picked up her speed and ran as fast as she could. He lunged toward her and picked her up by the throat. He punched her and pinned her down, trying to choke her. She felt her body detach as she screamed, "NO!" Her loud scream scared him off and he fled. Marie's whole body was shaking as she ran in the other direction to safety.*

Fortunately, Marie escaped from her attacker. Unfortunately, Marie experienced lasting effects from the event. Normal life occurrences now triggered that alarmed response she felt during the attack. One time she was putting money into a parking meter and a woman bumped into her. She completely panicked, her heart beating as if it would burst out of her chest. This reaction to benign events happened often. Whereas Marie used to look forward to her runs, her legs now turned to rubber every time she went out for one. She was afraid to run alone, even during the day. She got a dog, hoping it would make her feel safer at home and on the runs. What once used to bring her such joy and freedom was now a source of stress. Marie found herself getting inexplicable hives and frequently getting sick. Fear and anxiety were taking over her life.

The Mind quadrant represents our thoughts, emotions, memories, perceptions, and states of mind. Tending to the mind is important because what happens in the mind affects the body. Negative emotions such as anger, fear, guilt, worry, and loneliness can have a detrimental effect on the body, contributing to disease and illness. Positive emotions like joy, love, hope, and laughter can have a beneficial effect on the body, promoting health and healing.

The true story above illustrates the role that stress plays in our lives—for better or worse. Stress is a natural and highly adaptive biological process that strengthens and safeguards us in many ways. In the moment before Marie was attacked, she felt fear. In this case, fear was a good thing because it put her body in fight-or-flight mode. This is the body's classic sympathetic nervous system response to stress, which can save your life in an emergency. When a swift getaway or super strength is needed, stress is your body's call to action. For Marie, an increase in heart rate and blood pressure enabled her to be alert and respond in this situation by screaming, "NO!" which helped her get to safety.

Emotions like anger, fear, and worry are part of our way of navigating life. Problems arise when these emotions become a chronic state and begin to take a toll on our health. Marie experienced this by having hives and a lowered immune system. Once she got help, she was able to reclaim control of her life. She wore a whistle around her neck when she ran which gave her a sense of safety. She took comfort in recognizing that the fear she felt in that moment is what saved her. As she began to feel an increased sense of safety, she moved out of the constant state of fear and back into homeostasis (balance in her body).

Today, many of us live in a chronic state of stress, and it is making us sick. This state may have been initially triggered by an acute situation like Marie's and then lingered over time, or it can be from the continual stressors of life. Nearly 45% of all adults suffer adverse health effects due to stress, and 75 to 90% of all visits to primary care physicians are for stress-related complaints.[4] Long-term stress has been linked to high blood pressure, insomnia, ulcers, heart disease, diabetes, digestive system diseases, cancer, and aging.

The good news is that stress is not only what happens to us; it is also how we react to the stressors. Two people can be faced with the same stressful event and react differently. This means we have the power to manage our stress. If a woman cuts in front of you in line, your initial response might be to react by being angry and irritated. Instead, you can choose to use a coping strategy, such as reframing, by considering the possibility that she is not purposely being rude. Perhaps she just received some terrible news and is completely unaware that she cut in line. As discussed in *You're Laughing Now* and *What a Difference a Day Makes*, reframing is a way of changing the way you look at something to change your experience of it. You could also choose to try a relaxation technique to change your physiological response to stress. As discussed in *Meditation with Hollywood* and *Rise and Fall*, you can meditate and take breaths to calm yourself when you feel your body reacting to stress.

Our mental states can both promote health and encourage disease. You've probably heard of the placebo effect. A placebo is an inactive substance used in clinical testing of new drugs. Some of the patients in the trial are given the drug being tested while others (the control group) receive the inactive substance. The patients don't know if they're getting the real drug or the placebo. Amazingly, in numerous studies across a broad range of health issues, patients consistently experience relief from their symptoms even though they were given the placebo. This shows the power of the mind to heal the body. The patient believes the placebo is helping them heal, and so it does—not by the pill itself, but by the thoughts and beliefs in their minds. Placebos have been shown to increase hair growth in balding men, increase lung capacity in children with asthma, and provide pain relief equal to that of real knee surgery.[5]

There has even been research that a "nocebo" effect exists. This is when a negative health condition is caused by the expectation that one will develop that health condition. A great example is the Framingham Heart Study, in which thousands of residents of Framingham, Massachusetts, have been followed over decades. Women who believed they were prone to heart disease were nearly four times as likely to die from a heart attack as women with similar risk factors who did not have this fear.[6]

Not only can our positive thoughts help us heal, but also our negative thoughts can make us sick. Clearly the mind is an influential component of our health. It serves us well to have a mind that is happy, optimistic, and calm. There are many ways to nurture our mind (and reduce stress), in addition to the ones mentioned above. Additional topics covered in the following chapters include laughing, living mindfully, being authentic, and living proactively.

Read on to learn about changes you can make in your Mind to promote your overall health.

1

Creating Your Masterpiece

We are the artists of our own lives. We can create our own masterpieces. However, too often we focus on the daily challenges and end up on autopilot, letting our lives happen to us instead of leading the way. You have one life. Make it the one *you* want. As Confucius said, *"If we do not change our direction, we will end up where we are headed."* Is that where you want to go?

I spent the first four decades of my life searching—searching for my purpose, my passion, my place in this world. I once saw a greeting card with the quote, *"Not all who wander are lost"* by J.R.R. Tolkien. I bought the card and hung it in my office. It was a nice sentiment that I wanted to believe. Unfortunately, try as I might, it just didn't apply to me. I was wandering *and* I was lost.

I worked for over a decade in a career that was not authentically me. To the outside world, I was a "success." I was in a high paying job, working for a highly regarded company. The truth was, I was uncomfortable, unsettled, and unfulfilled. I had bursts of trying to find my way. I took numerous tests to figure out my "type" to help guide me. I know I am a Myers-Briggs ISTJ and an Enneagram 1. Unfortunately, this information did not bring me any closer to discovering my way. I looked into many different careers. At various points along the way, I thought I might want to be an event planner, franchise owner, therapist, entrepreneur, photographer, private detective, CIA agent, or geriatric counselor. I envied people who knew what they wanted to do from an early age.

I didn't know what I wanted to do and, even if I did, I was

committed to my career. After all, I had spent two years and a lot of money to get my MBA, and I had landed a highly coveted job out of school. The longer I stayed in the job, the more invested in it I became. I worried that if I left this line of work, my education and experience would be for nothing.

Throughout the years, I would often say to my husband, "I feel like I'm destined for more." I talked to him about all the things I could be doing, learning, and exploring. One day, he told me to stop talking and start doing. And so, I did. I took back control of my life. I left the corporate world. Simply being out of that environment paved the way for me to be the artist of my life again. I explored things that were of interest to me, rather than focusing on where the money was or what was desirable by society's standards. Even though I was still wandering, I no longer felt lost.

I wrote a list of areas I wanted to explore and started researching them one by one. Several items on the list led me to another masters program—this time studying holistic health education. Once I got off of autopilot and left behind what I thought I *should* be doing, I got out of my own way. This allowed me to proactively live the life I wanted to be living.

Do you feel like you are not creating the life you want? If so, it is time to get off autopilot, pick up the paintbrush, and start creating. Even if you feel stuck, realize that you *always* have choices. You may not be able to leave your job immediately, but you can make changes within your job to make it better. If the workload is too much, suggest ideas on what can be done more efficiently or ask for additional resources.

If that doesn't work, you always have a secret weapon: changing your mindset. Instead of focusing on what you don't like about your job, look at the benefits it provides you like flexibility to work from home so you have more time with the kids or money so you can take the trips you love. Own the fact that you are making the choice to stay in your job because of what it gives you. Reframing your mindset from I *have to* versus I *choose to* allows you to take back control of your life. This frees you to move from victim to creator.

Don't let yourself be a passive participant in the game of life. Have an active role in every situation you encounter—whether it is changing an aspect of your life or simply changing your mindset about it. As George Eliot, English Victorian novelist, said, *"It is never too late to be what you might have been."*

Who is painting the picture of your life? If it is not you, grab the paintbrush now and start creating your masterpiece.

2

Wish I Were Here

"Having a great time. Wish I were here." I saw this quote on a postcard a long time ago, and it always stuck with me. How often are you at a party, going about your daily life, or even on vacation without really being there? Perhaps you are still stuck in yesterday thinking about the argument you had with your spouse or maybe you are already in tomorrow worrying about your big presentation.

Living in the present sounds so simple, but is actually quite challenging. Ruminating about what happened in the past seems to come without effort, doesn't it? And, with so many demands on our time, it is hard not to be thinking about the future and all that needs to be done. How can we make it feel more natural to simply be in this moment?

Try living in the present right now. As you are reading this book, recognize that you are taking the time and reading a book. Notice where you are sitting, how your body is feeling, and what sounds you hear. Read the words on the page and just be in the moment of reading. You have decided to take time out to read this book, so try to be with it fully for the next few minutes. If you are doing other things in addition to reading this book—such as listening to music, watching TV, or eating—try doing just one thing, reading.

Mindfulness is about being conscious of the present moment in all that you do, filling your body's senses with what you are experiencing right now. Remember, you only have this moment once in your life. You might as well savor it by fully being with the activity you have decided to focus on. Try the *Now I Am Aware* exercise to help bring you in the present moment. How can you finish the sentence, "Now I am aware…"? For example:

Now I am aware…of the hum of the air cleaner.

Now I am aware…of a car driving by.

Now I am aware…of my dog chewing on a toy.

Now I am aware…of tightness in my neck.

Now I am aware…of an itch on my knee.

Now I am aware…of the sun streaming in the window.

Doing this exercise helps you become more present and aware of your senses—what you are seeing, feeling, and hearing in this moment. You can then take it one step further and allow yourself to *be* in your current activity exclusively. There are times in your life when this happens naturally because it is hard to be anywhere else. For example, when you are riding a roller coaster or skiing downhill, you are typically so absorbed in that activity that you are in the now. This can even happen in a movie theater. You can be so immersed in the movie that you don't hear the person next to you munching on popcorn or feel your knees stiffening up from sitting so long.

The challenge is to bring this presence to every day activities like washing the dishes, making the bed, walking the dog, or eating a meal. Starting with the *Now I Am Aware* exercise is a great first step to bring you into the present moment. Then allow yourself to simply *be.*

The beauty of mindfulness is that it can be done anywhere and anytime. The more we do it, the more we encourage health and wellness by breaking the cycle of the chronic state of stress that has become our daily lives.

In *The Power of Now*, Eckhart Tolle says that the present moment is where we find our joy and are able to embrace our true selves. He says it is here that we discover we are already complete and perfect. The beauty is that this is fully in reach for everyone. We just have to simply be. Here. Now.

Next time I'm having a great time, I plan to be there. How about you?

3

You're Laughing Now?

Over a decade ago, I was standing at baggage claim at the airport waiting for my luggage. There was a woman with three kids traveling alone, waiting for her luggage. She had her arms full with carry-on bags and her kids were running around. As she stood there, the bottom of the paper bag that she was holding ripped and all of the bag's contents dropped to the floor. I remember feeling empathy for her, knowing that if I had been in that situation, I would not have reacted well. How did she react?

Did she yell at her kids?

No.

Did she fly into a rage?

No.

Did she swear?

No.

Did she cry?

No.

She laughed.

To this day, I remember this woman and her reaction. It stands out in my mind because I would be challenged to handle this situation with such grace. Fortunately, I am married to a man who has a similar temperament to the woman at the airport. A few years back, we traveled to Northern Canada to see polar bears. We were flying out of Winnipeg and we were snowed in. I love traveling, but when it is time to go home, my mind is set on going home. Flexibility is not my strong suit.

Because of the conditions and scarcity of outbound flights, we were pushed back two days. I was upset and stressed. I wanted to go home. While my first reaction was to whine to anyone who would listen and scheme about how I could get out sooner (though there really was no hope), my husband, Dave, had a different impulse. He walked outside the airport doors and came back in with a small snowman he had made from the falling snow—the same snow that was preventing us from getting home.

This simple gesture reminded me to lighten up. There was nothing we could do, so why not make the most of it? I had a choice. I could be miserable for the next two mandatory days in Winnipeg or I could have fun. It reminded me of the woman in the airport. The bag broke. She could feel negative about it or she could laugh at the craziness of traveling alone with three kids.

When I recounted this story to my friend, Raoul, he shared an example of his own. During the time that Raoul was battling a rare form of non-Hodgkin's lymphoma, his wife, Monique, was developing a succession plan at work for top-level leadership in the company she worked for. Strewn about her home office were presentations, white papers, and books on succession planning. One day, Monique said to Raoul, "You are not allowed to die—or at least not the same year our 10-year old dogs die."

Raoul replied, "I should develop my own succession plan if I kick the bucket. Since we've been married almost 10 years, you would not be very good at dating, so let's figure out who will take my place. Tell me what you are looking for in your next husband and I'll start to do a search for you."

Raoul says that this conversation led to many laughs along the way during his eight-month battle with cancer. He would tease about what Monique was looking for and whether, like Raoul, he had to speak Spanish and love Greyhound dogs. Raoul said that the whole journey and how they handled it together brought them closer than they had ever been in their relationship. Death was staring them in the face and they chose to laugh. Fortunately, no succession plan was needed.

How we react to the stressors in our lives can absolutely affect our health. Studies show that people who have a positive outlook and feel a sense of control over their lives have been found to have fewer illnesses, fewer doctor visits, faster healing, improved survival after heart attacks, and improved cancer survival rates.

Learning from the examples above, here are five ways to find humor in stressful situations.

1. **Be objective.** Learning from the woman at the airport, she was able to step out of the craziness of the moment and see the situation objectively. Some women might have yelled at their kids to stop running around as if somehow that would have prevented the bag from ripping. It is a natural response to want some sense of control, but the bag ripping was no one's fault. The woman at the airport was able to see the humor in the mayhem that was happening around her, like she was a third party observer reading about this scenario in a Ziggy comic strip.

2. **Reframe the situation.** My husband was able to reframe the situation. Instead of feeling trapped and panicked because we had no control over getting out of Winnipeg, my husband chose to see it as an opportunity to have a few extra days of vacation, having fun in the snow.

3. **Let go of control.** The reason I was so upset in Winnipeg is because I had no control over getting home when I wanted. I was consumed with stress and anger. If I could have accepted the situation, let go of control, and moved forward,

I would have been more likely to see the fun in it. It's like the Serenity prayer says, *"Grant me the serenity to accept the things I cannot change; courage to change the things I can; and wisdom to know the difference."*

4. **Feel gratitude.** When you are grateful for what you have, it is hard to be angry or stressed. Instead of focusing on the negative, Raoul and Monique were grateful that Raoul was alive and getting treatment for his illness. If I could go back to that moment in Winnipeg, I would do it differently by trying to turn my stress into gratitude. I could have been grateful that the airlines were flying responsibly, putting safety first, and that I had more time on vacation with my husband.

5. **Lighten up.** Joking about the succession plan allowed Raoul and Monique to address a very serious concern—Raoul's possible death. Bringing lightness to a situation does not minimize the seriousness of it. Sometimes it makes it more accessible and manageable. As mentioned in the chapter, *Birthday Hat Dare,* laughter counteracts the effects of stress physiologically in the body, so joking about the succession plan was one of the healthiest things Raoul and Monique could do for themselves.

I haven't mastered the art of finding humor in typically stressful situations, but I'm working on it. Think about a past stressful situation. How could humor have lightened your load?

4

Meditation with Hollywood

When you think of meditation, you probably think of sitting in a lotus position repeating the mantra, "om." For years, meditation has been on my to-do list. I have tried to meditate at various points in my life, but my mind wandered and I was uncomfortable in the recommended sitting position. When I focused on my breath, I didn't seem to be breathing comfortably. Because of my preconceived notion of what it meant to meditate, I felt like a failure at it.

One morning as I was lying in bed with my cat, Hollywood, having our morning snuggle time, I realized that this is my meditation. While Hollywood is on me or next to me, my mind is quiet and I am focused only on him and the connection between us. I pay attention to the feel of his fur, the closing of his eyes, and the purr of his body. His purr is the vibration of his happiness and I let it permeate my being. During the meditation, I feel my mind clear and my body relax. My breath slows, my heart rate lowers, and I feel calm. This happens without me even thinking about it. Sometimes I'm there for five minutes and sometimes for twenty. My meditation is simple, and I am good at it—just the way it should be.

Is your meditation practice more traditional, sitting in the lotus position and focusing on your breath or repeating a mantra? Or is it something a little less traditional, like staring at the ocean, sitting in your recliner chair and listening to music, walking along the beach, or working in the garden? Whatever it is, try to clear your mind and passively focus on one thing—whether it be your breath, a word, your cat's purr, the sound of the waves, or the feel of dirt in your fingers.

Meditation is about creating space in your mind, quieting the incessant mental chatter. If thoughts come up, it's okay. Bring yourself back to your quiet mind without judgment or frustration. Try to be a third party observer of your thoughts, without taking a personal interest in them. Meditate in a place where the distractions are limited. You want to be grounded in the silence and stillness of present moment awareness.

If meditating feels like work, you are trying too hard. Meditating should come easily and calmly, which is why it is so important to find the way that works for you. We are all so busy in our lives *doing*. Meditation is about taking a few moments and simply *being*. It is amazing what rejuvenation can come from just a few minutes of quieting the mind.

Meditation has been shown to be helpful in both disease prevention and health promotion. Studies show numerous physiological and psychological benefits of meditation. Some of the physiological benefits include lower blood pressure, strengthened immune system, relaxed muscles, and improved digestion. Psychological benefits include decreased anxiety and depression, increased productivity, and improved memory.

Is there an activity that you enjoy doing that you now realize is your form of meditation? If so, how can you incorporate it more into your daily life?

5

Productive Unproductiveness

Sitting by the fire in your pajamas at noon reading a book may seem like a luxury, but actually it can be essential for your health. You know that feeling when you aren't fully engaging in life, even the simplest things seem overwhelming, and you are extra sensitive to people's comments and behavior? That's when it's time for some productive unproductiveness.

Research has been done on the relationship between stress and productivity. The Human Function Curve, as shown below, depicts this relationship. It is illustrated graphically as an upside down letter U. As stress increases (the horizontal axis), so does productivity (the vertical axis)—illustrated by the light gray, upward sloping portion of the curve. At a point, the positive relationship ends—represented by the top of the curve and the limit line. After that, as stress increases, productivity decreases—shown by the dark gray, downward sloping portion of the curve. When you get in this zone, exhaustion and burnout occur. This ultimately leads to illness. If you find yourself reaching the limit line, it's time for a break.

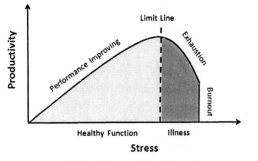

The Human Function Curve

Another way to think about this is to imagine that your stress level is like the RPM on a car's tachometer. In order for your car to run optimally and to prevent engine failure, you want to keep the indicator below the red zone. When your car is being revved too high, you can hear it being overtaxed. As soon as you shift into a different gear, it quiets down and runs smoothly.

Have you experienced this—where you are so busy and you know you should slow down because you are running yourself ragged, but you don't because there is so much to do? Then you end up getting sick and you have no choice but to relax. The rest required for recovery once you hit the limit line is even more than needed before hitting the line, so in the end, you end up losing productivity. To top it all off, you aren't even able to enjoy the rest time at that point because you feel lousy.

If there is a time when you feel like you are hitting the limit line or getting into the RPM red zone, don't try to justify or rationalize it. Acknowledge it and take the steps that work for you to get some rest. You not only deserve it, it's necessary for you to move forward productively. You cannot function fully without taking a break. Can you take a day off from work? If not a full day, how about a morning or afternoon? Even an hour can do wonders.

Think about what brings you back into the healthy function zone. Perhaps it's taking a walk, reading a good book, snuggling with your pet, or getting a massage. Or maybe it's working on a jigsaw puzzle, watching reruns of your favorite TV show, staying in bed an extra hour, or meeting a friend for lunch.

As Scarlett O'Hara says in *Gone with the Wind*, *"Tomorrow is another day."* Yes, it is. So, when you are feeling tired and overwhelmed by the simplest tasks, let tomorrow be the day for the tasks and today be the day for you.

Next time you are close to hitting the limit line, how will you engage in some productive unproductiveness?

6

Free to Be Me

It has taken me 40 years to figure out that being authentic is the best thing I can do for my health and well-being. I find that it actually takes work and causes me stress when I am *not* being true to myself. Medieval mystic, Mechthild of Magdeburg, said, "*A fish cannot drown in water. A bird does not fall in air. Each creature God made must live in its own true nature.*" When we struggle to fit a false image, we fall or drown. When we are true to our nature, we boundlessly thrive.

Recently I got together with a few friends from business school that I hadn't seen in almost 18 years. The next day, one of the friends said to me, "They all said you were glowing. Why do you think you glow?"

I replied, "I glow because I am living authentically!"

Living true to yourself means following your own path despite what others are doing. It means not trying to be someone you are not in order to please others. It is easy to get caught up in what you think you should do, what society expects from you, or what your friends want you to do. This can take many forms—including how you eat, exercise, make your living, and spend your free time.

Here are nine tips for living authentically that have helped me find my way:

1. **Know your purpose.** Life becomes so much more meaningful when we have a purpose that is tied to who we are. It makes us want to get out of bed in the morning and

contribute to the world around us. Knowing your purpose helps you weather the storms of life so that you stay on course. You can always find your way back by returning to your purpose.

I now know that my purpose is to help others create more health in their lives. Staying true to this has led me to a career that energizes rather than drains me.

2. **Live *in the flow*.** *The flow* is a powerful state of being where life seems to be moving effortlessly. You feel relaxed and present. You feel completely absorbed by the task at hand. Hours go by without recognition—often filled with high creativity and productivity. Think about times when you experience this feeling. It could be when you are engaging in sports, playing a musical instrument, putting together a scrapbook, gardening, or doing a certain project at work. Be sure to bring these activities into your life as often as you can.

For me, when I am writing, I feel *in the flow*. Hours pass by when I am writing. I become completely absorbed with typing the words on the page, placing them exactly where I want them in order to convey my message. Spending more time *in the flow* makes me happier and allows me to give my best self to the world.

3. **Quiet your mind.** Find your meditation, as described in the chapter, *Meditation with Hollywood*, in order to take a few moments every day to quiet the mental chatter in your mind. Some of us are afraid of the silence and others don't value it. We tend to fill our days to the max. Even when we do have down time, we often choose to watch television instead of sitting quietly and allowing our minds to rest.

Quieting the mind allows you to sort through the noise and get back to being true to yourself.

My mind is not naturally quiet, so this practice has been very helpful in giving me a break from the ticker tape running constantly in my mind. Often times I get clarity on a situation, and I always feel rejuvenated.

4. **Focus on the positive.** Try to see the positive flipside of the things you don't like about yourself. For example, if you feel that you are not flexible enough, realize that this could be the flipside of being such a good planner. Give yourself plenty of self-love and appreciate yourself just the way you are.

Focusing on the positive allowed me to reach my full potential, without the doubts and self-bashing getting in the way. I am someone who does not think fast on my feet. I am more of a processor. I used to feel inadequate in business meetings when discussing a new topic. Then I realized that my moment to shine is after the meeting when I have had time to process. I have a talent for taking what I hear in a meeting, synthesizing it, and coming up with well-thought out ideas. Knowing my strengths allows me to better set myself up for success so that I feel good, not bad, about myself.

5. **Choose your friends wisely.** Not only do you need to appreciate yourself just the way you are, but also you need to surround yourself with others who do too. Doing otherwise can be a serious impediment to living authentically. Think about what it feels like when someone loves you for exactly who you are, quirks and all. You don't have to pretend to be someone you are not. You want people who love you not *in*

spite of who you are, but *because of* who you are.

I am done spending time not being myself in order to fit in with others. Instead, I surround myself with people who lift me up and who share my interests. This is discussed in the chapters, *Exiting Stage Left* and *Find Your People*, found in Part Three, the Relationships quadrant.

6. **Don't be afraid of failure.** As highlighted in the upcoming chapter, *If You Knew You Could Not Fail*, we can accomplish amazing feats and be our full selves when we take the fear of failure out of the equation. Don't let the fear stop you from following your authentic path and being the largest version of you.

I used to let the fear of failure prevent me from trying new things. By learning to reframe the concept of failure, I have taken away its power. As Thomas Edison said, *"I have not failed, just found 10,000 ways that won't work."*

7. **Trust your inner guide.** You know what is right for you. You simply need to be open enough to hear it and courageous enough to listen and act. When something doesn't feel right, trust that instinct. Don't let anyone talk you out of trusting the gut feeling you have.

It really works. When I listen to my inner wisdom, I find that I have the answers. If it doesn't feel right, I don't do it.

8. **Declare yourself.** Boldly say who you are and who you want to be. At first, I felt shy about calling myself a writer because I was new at it, but then I came across a wonderful quote from an artist named Faith Ringgold. Ringgold says, "Back when I was starting out, someone at a party asked me what I did, and I said, 'I'm an artist.' A friend of mine said, 'Faith,

would you please stop telling people you're an artist? You're not an artist. You're an art teacher.' I thought: That's interesting that she thinks she can tell me who I am. I'm the one who determines when I'm an artist. And that's right here, right now."

I love this idea of declaring who we are and who we want to be. Faith Ringgold is an artist. I am a writer. Who are you?

9. **Let go of ego.** Don't let societal beliefs and standards influence your way. It is hard to venture on a path that friends and family might not understand, but they will understand when they see you thriving in all of your authentic glory.

My ego was one of the primary reasons I stayed in an unfulfilling career for 10 years. I let what others considered success and the right path drive my direction. When I let go of my ego, it freed me up to find my way.

Embrace the fact that you are unique. No one is exactly like you, which means that what is authentic for you may not be what is right for someone else. And, what is right for someone else may not be right for you. As Judy Garland said, *"Always be a first-rate version of yourself, instead of a second-rate version of somebody else."* Be you. Nobody does it better.

Do you feel free to be you? If not, what steps can you take to feel that freedom?

7

Birthday Hat Dare

What is free, fun, and good for your health? Laughter. Yet, how many times a day do you find yourself laughing?

There have been numerous studies done on the effects of laughter on our health. In fact, Greeks, ancient Africans, American Indians, and medieval European kings and queens have used humor in healing for over 2,000 years. The research shows that there are both short-term and long-term physiological effects when we laugh. Laughter has been credited with lowering blood pressure, improving circulatory and cardiovascular health, facilitating digestion, and boosting the immune system. Two stress hormones, epinephrine and cortisol, drop after a healthy dose of laughter which means laughter is a great counterbalance to stress.

How can you get more laughter and fun into your life? The birthday hat dare is certainly one way. As my friends and family know, I have a thing about birthday hats. When it is my birthday, I wear a birthday hat no matter what I am doing that day. I have worn hats in movie theaters, at restaurants, walking the streets of San Francisco, running trails, and strolling the Santa Cruz boardwalk.

All those who share my special day with me are subjected to wearing hats too. I love seeing other people smile as they go by us. How often are adults walking around wearing birthday hats? Plus, who doesn't love the extra "happy birthday" greetings from complete strangers?

My husband, Dave, who some might say is more on the

reserved side, took the birthday hat wearing to a whole new level this year. On his birthday, Dave had to travel to Birmingham, Alabama, for business. He wore a birthday hat from the moment he left our house in the morning to the time he went to bed in Birmingham that night. This included wearing the hat through airport security in Oakland, California, on the plane, during a plane change in Phoenix, Arizona, in the cab to the hotel, and checking in at the hotel. He was invited into the cockpit on both flights, had an entire plane of people sing Happy Birthday to him, and was offered a free beer at his hotel. He wasn't even traveling with colleagues; he was traveling alone!

On your next birthday, I dare you to wear a birthday hat for at least part of the day. If your birthday is not for another few months, put a reminder on the calendar right now on your special day that says "birthday hat dare."

Since your birthday only comes once a year, think about other ways to laugh more often, like hula hooping. We bought hula hoops for my birthday party last year. They were a hit and definitely had us laughing. Other ideas could be to play a game like charades, watch stand-up comedy, or have a joke-telling contest.

Laughing is not simply something fun to do; it is good for your health. As Benjamin Franklin said, *"We do not stop playing because we grow old, we grow old because we stop playing."*

How can you have more fun and laughter in your life to bring up your daily giggle quota?

8

Rise and Fall

What is an extremely effective way to reduce stress that is free, easy, and portable—and with you your entire life? Breathing!

The next time you feel your stress level rising, take a time out and breathe. You can do it anywhere, anytime—at work, while waiting in line at the grocery store or doctor's office, or before bed. You can do it while sitting, lying down, and even walking.

We breathe about 20,000 times a day. We might as well be doing it the optimal way that promotes health. In a normal resting state, the average person breathes in and out about 14 to 16 times per minute. Under stress, this can increase to nearly 30 and in a deeply relaxed state it can be as low as five.

When we are under stress, our breathing tends to be quick and shallow, using the top half of the lungs. This shallow breathing sends a message to our body that we are in fight-or-flight mode and we begin to pump out stress hormones. These stress hormones can suppress the cells of our immune system, leaving us more susceptible to illness.

The breathing style that produces the greatest relaxation response is that which allows the stomach to expand rather than the upper chest. This is actually how we breathe when we are comfortably asleep and how we breathed when we were babies. It is known as diaphragmatic or belly breathing. Breathing this way allows for maximal oxygen intake and carbon dioxide release. Many of the effects of belly breathing are the opposite of the effects of stress. For example, the simple act of deep breathing can calm the nervous system, lower the heart rate, reduce blood pressure, and improve the digestive process—all of which promote our health and well-being.

The following four steps will guide you to breathe deeply:

1. **Sit comfortably** with your back straight. Put one hand on your chest and the other hand on your stomach.

2. **Breathe in** through your nose. The hand on your stomach should rise. The hand on your chest should move very little.

3. **Exhale out** through your mouth, pushing out as much air as you can while contracting your abdominal muscles. The hand on your stomach should move in as you exhale, but the hand on your chest should not move very much.

4. **Continue to breathe** in through your nose and out through your mouth. In a few deep breaths, you will feel calmer and more relaxed.

Some people like to count with each exhalation, thinking of nothing but the number as they breathe in and out. Others like to say a mantra as they breathe in and out. For example, "I breathe in peace (calm, health, joy, trust) and I breathe out fear (anger, insecurity, stress)." Some simply like to follow the rise and fall of their breath.

A teacher of mine used to say, "Show me how you breathe and I will tell you how you live." My breath tends to be shallow and quick because I'm a Type A, on-the-go, worrier kind of gal. I need to actively work on slowing down and breathing deeper. My husband, Dave, who is a laid back, it-will-all-work-out, kind of guy naturally has a slower and deeper breathing pattern.

Pay attention to your breath now. What is it saying about you and your life?

9

Losing My Mind(fulness)

Are you so busy that you are losing your mind(fulness)? The other day I forgot to put eggs in the water for my morning hard-boiled eggs. I returned to the stove 15 minutes later to find a pot of boiling water. A friend said she forgot to pick up her kids from school. A client said he completely missed an appointment that was clearly marked on his calendar. I'm sure we all have our stories of what happens when we become mindlessly busy.

When we get to this point, we often end up creating even more work for ourselves. One time, I was supposed to pick up my friend, Christy, to take her to catch the train to the airport. She texted me 10 minutes after I was supposed to pick her up asking me if I was on my way. Nope, I wasn't. I was working at home with a million things on my mind and a long to-do list for the day. Despite the fact that she had only asked me two days prior, and it was on my calendar, I had no recollection of this important pending appointment.

I flew out of my house and ended up having to make the hour drive each way to the airport because it was too late for her to take the train and make her flight. What would have been a 30-minute diversion from my packed day became a two-hour time commitment. Do you see the irony? My busyness actually took time away from me. I was so busy that I was losing my mindfulness.

We all have so many demands on our time and so many things to get done in a day. How can we manage it all and still keep our sanity? Try taking five minutes at the beginning of every day, whether it's while lying in bed, drinking a cup of tea, or sitting in your yard. During the five minutes, try to do these five things.

1. **Review your schedule for the coming day.** Reviewing your schedule is useful so that your commitments are fresh in your mind for the day.

2. **Take a few deep breaths.** As covered in the last chapter, *Rise and Fall*, breathing is a powerful and effective way to promote your health and wellness.

3. **Be grateful.** Taking a moment in the morning to be grateful is a good reminder of all of the wonderful things in your life and sets a positive, loving tone for the day. What are you grateful for? Perhaps today you are grateful for the friends and family in your life. Tomorrow it may be the sunshine, a good book, or the smell of a rose.

4. **Set your intention.** Setting an intention gives energy and focus to the day. Ideas for intention include being mindful, grateful, open, strong, productive, playful, healthy, and happy. Wake up every morning with the expectation of having a great day.

5. **Meditate (Just be).** Taking a moment to meditate allows you to have at least a few minutes in your hectic day to enjoy a quiet moment. As discussed in *Meditation with Hollywood*, "meditation" comes in many forms and it's about finding your own way of clearing your mind. You may not have time during this morning ritual to listen to music or feel your cat's purr. Even simply taking time at the breakfast table, feeling the warmth of your hot cup of

tea and just "being" will work. Remember, it's about grounding yourself in the silence and stillness of present moment awareness—even if only for a minute or two.

I'm busy, but not so busy that I can't take five minutes of every day to begin it properly. And, for those really important appointments, I now set a pop-up reminder on my online calendar.

What changes can you make so that you don't lose your mind(fulness)?

10

What a Difference a Day Makes

"**W**hat a difference a day makes." This was my sister's mantra as she battled Stage 3 breast cancer for over a year. I think of this mantra often because it applies to all of us—no matter what challenge we are facing in our lives.

When Debbie was going through treatment, which included chemotherapy, stem cell transplant, surgery, and radiation, she had good days, and she had bad days. What got her through the bad days was knowing that there would be good days. She knew that even though she might feel really bad today, it didn't mean that was how she would feel tomorrow or the next day. A jingle used commercially for C&R Clothiers kept playing in her head.

What a difference a day makes
Twenty-four little hours
What a difference a day makes
And the difference is you

I did some research and found out that the jingle came from a song, *What a Difference a Day Makes*, that was popular in the 1950s and sung by Dinah Washington. Knowing how much her mantra inspired her to get through the bad days, I bought her the CD. Debbie would listen to the song over and over again, as many times as she needed to get through the low days.

Are you going through a tough time right now? Do you have a health issue of your own or have you experienced a loss? Are you going through a life change or having trouble in a relationship? Are you a new mom exhausted from lack of sleep? It may not even be one large event that is bringing you down, but rather the accumulation of many little things.

When something bad happens to us, we get brought down and can feel overwhelmed by the news or experience. Here are eight tips for helping yourself feel better during the hard times.

1. **Be a third person observer of your life.** If you are feeling low because you are going through a divorce, try saying to yourself, "So this is what it feels like to be going through a divorce." Identify how it is making you feel. "It is making me feel anxious and I feel my heart racing. I find myself snapping at everyone because I am feeling angry and hurt from the divorce." By being able to identify and objectify your feelings, it helps to keep you detached and out of the whirlwind of despair.

2. **Remember the difference is you.** A key part of the jingle is, "the difference is you." There may be a lot about your situation that is not in your control, but focusing on the things that are in your control helps to empower you. As discussed in *You're Laughing Now?*, you can do so by finding humor in the situation, being grateful for what you do have, and reframing the situation. You can also try smiling, which sends a signal to your brain that everything is okay.

3. **Don't be defined by the situation.** If you have been diagnosed with cancer, don't see yourself only as a cancer patient. If your marriage recently ended or you were laid off, don't merely think of yourself as a divorcee or as someone who is unemployed. Focus on the parts of your life that bring you joy. Remind yourself of who you are outside of the illness or situation.

4. **Be kind and true to yourself.** Take the time to nurture yourself during the hard times. Don't feel like you have to be super-person and be strong for everyone else. Honor where you are at and be okay with it.

5. **Ask for help.** Many of my clients are afraid to ask for help. They say they don't want to be seen as emotionally weak. Allowing yourself to be vulnerable with others is a great way to form intimate bonds. If you share your feelings with others when you are down, it helps them to feel comfortable to do so when they are down. Your friends and family want to help you. Let them.

6. **Mourn the loss.** When you first find out about an illness, lose a loved one, get laid off, or experience any other life-changing event, it is important to take the time to mourn the loss of your old life. This can also apply to happy events like having a baby, moving to a new house, or changing jobs. Recognizing that your life will not be the same and mourning the loss of what was allows you to let go and move forward. Without taking this step, you remain stuck, longing for the way things were. Be open to your new life. It will be different, but new sources of happiness and joy await you.

7. **Discover the stars.** There is a Persian proverb: *"When it is dark enough, you can see the stars."* Sometimes in our darkest hour, we are enlightened by an idea or a new way of being. When we are stripped down to our most raw and vulnerable self, we often see what and who is truly important to us. This unexpected and unrequested gift from a difficult time

may not come right away, but try to be open to and accepting of it when it arrives.

8. **Take a four quadrant perspective.** Focus on creating health in the areas where you can. If you have a physical illness, you have the choice of whether you let it affect you in the other three quadrants of your life. This point is illustrated further in the following chapter, *The Mental in Illness.* One of my clients let a hip injury negatively impact her mind, relationships, and environment. If she had chosen to nurture these areas instead, she would have been a lot healthier and happier—even with her physical injury.

On days when you are feeling overwhelmed, remember that not every day is going to be like this. In fact, the bad days will start to come farther apart. They did for my sister and they will for you too.

Are you having a bad day today? If so, remember what a difference a day makes.

11

The Mental in Illness

Do you think you are healthy? Believe it or not, the answer to this question can actually impact how healthy you really are. Research has shown that people who believed they were in poor health were three to six times more likely to die in the studied time period than those who believed they were in good health.[7]

Just because you have an illness does not automatically mean you are unhealthy. It can be *if you let it be*, but it doesn't have to be if you focus on creating health in the areas where you can. My client, Susan, has a hip injury. She has chronic pain and cannot stand for long periods of time. She tires easily.

Without a doubt, this would get anyone down, but Susan has let her physical illness define her. It completely consumes who she is. In one of our sessions together, she said, "I am an invalid." She has brought the mental into her physical illness and it is making her unhealthy.

Susan has let her illness impact all four quadrants of her life. In the Body quadrant where the illness resides (physical pain and immobility), she has let it impact her diet and movement. She eats a lot of packaged and fast foods. She doesn't get as much movement as she could, even with her physical limitations.

In the Mind quadrant, she has lost her zest for life. She sees herself as an invalid. When I ask her about a baseball game she went to recently with her family, she tells me about how tiring it was for her to sit for that long of a time. She doesn't tell me whether or not she enjoyed the game. It is all about the illness.

In the Relationships quadrant, she brings illness energy in to her social connections. Any time her friends, children, or husband try to get her to go out and engage with life again, she responds negatively. Susan spends most of her conversations with others talking about her illness.

In the Environment quadrant, her world has become very small. I suggested sitting outside in the warm sun. Instead of seeing the positive of this activity, she focused on the difficulty of making it down the few steps to get there. It is no longer as easy to sit outside, but she *can* do it. She *chooses* not to.

Susan can get the mental out of her illness by creating health in the areas where she can. She may not have control over some of what is happening in the Body quadrant because of her physical limitations, but she can eat healthier foods. This will bring her energy level up and keep her weight down. She can exercise those parts of her body that are not physically impaired like her upper body.

For her Mind, she can do visualizations or repeat mantras to help get her enthusiasm for life back. She can reframe how she looks at things. For example, instead of seeing herself as an invalid with so many limitations, she can see all that she still can do like going to the ball game with her family. It may wipe her out for the day, but she can work to slowly build up her strength and stamina. She can still enjoy cooking by inviting a friend over while they do the preparation and she guides the way. She may not be able to do some of the things that she used to do like play tennis, but she can find new areas of interest that fit her (temporary) sedentary lifestyle such as joining a book club, building puzzles, or knitting.

For her Relationships, Susan can focus on others rather than on herself. By engaging in new activities, Susan will have topics other than her illness to talk about with her loved ones. She will begin to feel better by not focusing on her illness 24/7. I challenged Susan for one week to not talk about her illness when she was with her friends and family. If they asked her how she was doing, I suggested she say that she was feeling better. Even if her immobility and pain level were the same, this could be a true statement if she improved her diet, increased her movement, and changed her mindset.

For the Environment, Susan could sit outside and enjoy nature. Even if she can't make it outside, sitting by a window and looking out is a great option.

Over the course of a few months, Susan worked on nourishing health in the areas of her life where she could affect change. Not surprisingly, she began to feel better, despite the fact that her physical limitations were the same. It wasn't until a year later that her hip pain subsided, but by then she had already chosen health over illness.

Susan is not alone. I've seen this with many clients where the mental seeps into their illness. Sometimes the mental lingers even after the physical illness is gone. That's how powerful a hold it can have. My client, Denise, had experienced months where she would get so lightheaded when she went out to dinner that she would have to leave restaurants abruptly, afraid she was going to pass out. Once she was diagnosed as prediabetic and got her blood sugar under control, she did not have the physical symptoms anymore. However, she would work herself into such a state worrying about it happening again, that she was afraid to go out to dinner. It took her a few more months to get the mental out of her illness and feel comfortable to go out to a restaurant again.

If you have an illness that is unnecessarily creeping into other areas of your life and bringing you down, try to recognize the role that your mind plays in the healing process and take steps to create health in the areas you can.

Do you think you are healthy? Let me hear a resounding, "Yes!" Remember, how you *perceive* your health can actually impact your health.

12

If You Knew You Could Not Fail

The question, "What would you do if you knew you could not fail?" changed my life. I came across it in a book about taking stock of who you are and what you want to do. The question was one among many. I wrote my responses to the questions in 2003 and 2005 without comparing my answers ahead of time. Both times I wrote, "run a marathon" in answer to this particular question. My response seemed odd considering I wasn't a runner and didn't even like running.

Despite having no interest in running, whenever I would meet someone who had run a marathon, I would be in complete and total awe. To me, it was an impossible goal. Given that I had written the same answer twice, I decided that running a marathon must be something I needed to do.

I began my journey with an online visit to Amazon and ordered a few books on how to run a marathon. In March of 2005, my first day of training consisted of alternating a five-minute run and a five-minute walk for 30 minutes. Seven months later, I had run over 530 miles. On October 23, 2005, I crossed the finish line of my first marathon.

For the first time in my life, I was to-the-core proud of myself. Yes, I had had academic and professional successes in my life, but excelling in these areas was in my comfort zone. Running marathons required me to push myself mentally and physically like I never had.

My husband told me after the marathon that one of my friends had asked him what we would do about the planned celebration party if I had not been able to finish the race. Honestly, it had never crossed my mind that I wouldn't finish the marathon. After all, the question that inspired me to run the marathon said I would not fail. I had set out to do it, and I would do it.

I didn't stop at one marathon. I was hooked on the high. To date, I've run six of them. At my third marathon, I wanted to quality for the Boston Marathon, the granddaddy of them all. To do so, I needed to run a marathon in 3 hours and 45 minutes. I wanted a 3:43 for cushion. I printed this number in large font and stuck it on my computer where I saw it every day during the four months of training. Despite needing to shave off over 20 minutes of my previous time, I set this lofty goal. I visualized the race from start to finish many times. Mentally, I had already run the marathon in 3:43. On race day, I just had to physically do it. I did. The finish time on the clock was 3:43. Setting your mind on a goal and visualizing the end result are powerful forces to be reckoned with.

My friend Darren is a perfect example of this powerful force. He hiked up (and down) all 4,800 feet of Half Dome in Yosemite with his mind. His body followed. During training, Darren had struggled on every hike we did that had hills. On the day of the climb, Darren's stomach was bothering him from the first mile. He was unable to eat or drink anything without feeling sick. After staying with Darren for six of the eight miles to the top, the five of us in the group realized that Darren would not be making it to the top of Half Dome that day. We needed to make it up and down before nightfall, so we left him and continued on ourselves. We suggested he turn around and start making his way back down. We would catch up to him on our descent.

After we had enjoyed our time on the summit and were heading back down, we saw Darren climbing up the cables, the final step of making it to the top of the mountain. I have chills remembering this in my mind. Darren inspired me that day. Physically, there is no logical way that he should have been able to make it to the top. He had no food in him, he was hurting from the first mile, and he had no successful hilly training hikes. There is no doubt that he hiked 16 miles for 12 hours that day solely fueled by the power of his mind. He had such drive to make it to the top that there was no other option for the day.

On the top of the mountain, Darren shared with us that someone at his office had recently tried to climb Half Dome and had been unable to. This coworker told Darren he had to do it as the representative of the company. The coworker also spread the word in the office about Darren's endeavor, so in the weeks leading up to the hike, Darren had people asking him about it daily. They were all cheering him on. The day before the hike, Darren bought an "I climbed Half Dome" shirt in anticipation of reaching his goal the next day. One of the other people in our group said he would not buy the shirt until after he had actually done it. I think it's absolutely essential to buy the shirt beforehand. State your intention. Put your goal out there. Visualize getting it done. And then complete your goal. Say it. See it. Do it.

Eleven words put together to form such a powerful question: *What would you do if you knew you could not fail?* For me, these words gave me the gift of running and made me realize that I can do anything I set my mind to. I know Darren's experience changed his life too.

For my first marathon party, I asked everyone to write on a post-it note and put it on the wall of how they would answer the question. I still have those post-its. My dad wrote, "Be a concert pianist." My friend, Cecile, said, "Become fluent in French and live in Paris for a few years." My stepmom dreamed, "Be able to paint or draw and like the results."

What about you? What would you put on your post-it if you knew you could not fail?

Is Your Mind Healthy?

Indicators for health and illness in the Mind quadrant focus on our mental and emotional health. Thoughts, feelings, and emotions can affect our health. A "yes" answer represents an indicator for health and a "no" for illness, unless otherwise noted.

- Do you have a positive outlook on life?
- Are you happy?
- Do you think you deserve to be happy?
- Are you in control of your emotions?
- Do you express your feelings?
- Do you feel physically healthy?
- Do you feel emotionally healthy?
- Do you have laughter and fun in your life?
- Do you have a spiritual influence in your life?
- Do you have and enjoy time alone?
- Do you regularly engage in activities that bring you joy?
- Do you have hope?
- Are you able to forgive yourself and others?
- Are you living authentically?
- Do you have a positive self-image?
- Do you have a daily meditation practice?
- Do you look forward to waking up each day?
- Do you live in the present moment?
- Do you feel in control of your life?
- Do you feel engaged in your life?
- Do you allow yourself to have "me time"?
- Do you have a creative outlet?
- Do you rest when your mind is tired?

- Do you love yourself?
- Do you express gratitude?
- Do you spend time in nature?
- Do you have purpose in your life?
- Do you have work satisfaction?
- Do you feel stressed, anxious, or fearful? ("yes" is illness indicator)
- Do you feel angry, hurt, or resentful? ("yes" is illness indicator)
- Do you feel overwhelmed with life and responsibilities? ("yes" is illness indicator)
- Do you obsess about the past and/or worry about the future? ("yes" is illness indicator)
- Do you feel depressed, hopeless, and/or helpless? ("yes" is illness indicator)

Guided by the ideas in this section, look at where you answered "no" in the earlier questions and try to identify how these can become "yes." Do the same for the last five questions if you answered "yes" and try to figure out how they can become "no."

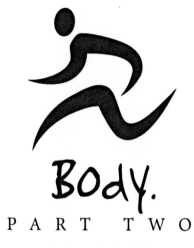

BODY.

P A R T   T W O

Body and Health

*B*ill *can't remember the last time he had a moment to himself. His life has become so busy since the children were born. In order to get everything done in a day, Bill finds himself getting less than six hours of sleep a night. He has two young boys, Zach and Ryan. His wife is always telling him he's not helping her enough with the kids, but he doesn't know how to find more time in the day. He feels stressed by the financial pressure of raising a family and saving money for the boys' college educations. Fortunately, his company is growing, but it means extra work for him.*

Bill has a lot of meetings with clients, so he eats out often. He never has time for swimming anymore. By the time he gets home, he's exhausted. The first thing he does when he gets home is pour himself a drink to help unwind. Over the years, Bill has gained weight steadily. When Bill went in for his annual checkup and blood work, he was shocked to learn that he weighed 40 pounds more than he did a few years prior. He was even more alarmed to find out that his cholesterol and triglycerides were high and he was prediabetic.

The Body quadrant represents our physical being. This quadrant is probably the one you are most familiar with in terms of health. Everywhere in the media, we see information about the benefits of eating right, exercising more, and sleeping well. We are reminded that when we aren't doing enough of these things, we hurt our health.

If you change a few of the details to the story above, does it resemble your life? Bill's story likely resonates with many people—both men and women. Bill's way of life for the past few years has finally caught up with him. He found himself eating out a lot with clients so he was overeating and not making healthy choices. He was eating a lot of fast foods and sweets too. He was self-medicating with his nightly glass (or two) of wine. He always felt exhausted when the alarm went off at six, but there was work to be done. His poor eating habits, lack of exercise, and other lifestyle choices showed up as 40 extra pounds, high cholesterol, and prediabetes.

Diet and exercise are the two elements of the Body quadrant that we hear about the most. Numerous studies show that eating a diet filled with processed foods, unhealthy fats, and refined sugars leads to health problems such as diabetes, heart disease, obesity, osteoarthritis, and cancer. Research shows the flipside to be true too—eating a nutritional diet can help prevent those same health problems.

In today's world, there is a lot of emphasis on "dieting" with the goal of losing weight. There are numerous weight loss programs promoting the latest shake, supplement, pill, plan, or product that you can buy to help shed those extra pounds. I have seen many clients who say they have tried most every product on the market. Some of the plans work for some individuals in the short term, but none of them work for anyone in the long term.

Because nutrition is such an important part of your health,

there are several chapters in this section about eating well. These chapters support healthy eating as a way of life, not as a quick fix for the short term. *Living in the 80s* provides some tips for following the 80/20 rule—eating healthy 80% of the time and mindfully indulging the other 20%. *Keeping it Real* underscores the importance of eating real food and educates you on reading labels. *The Trendy Diet* illustrates the role that the media play in our infatuation with the latest nutrition fads. *Fad Free Eating* gives you the top tips for eating healthy that will stand the test of time.

Exercise has also been shown to be an important influencer on health—both beneficial (when you do it) and harmful (when you don't). Benefits of exercise include decreases in resting heart rate, blood pressure, muscle tension, cholesterol, body fat, and stress. It also increases resistance to colds and illness, efficiency of the heart, sleep quality, energy, brain function, and longevity. The consequences of not doing it include diabetes, heart disease, depression, obesity, and more. These are some pretty good reasons to get up and move!

Our lives have become more sedentary than they were for our ancestors. For most of evolutionary history, humans didn't need to think about getting "exercise." Just living meant getting movement in life—whether we were walking, building a fire, making our clothes, hunting, or gathering. Today we have cars, elevators, food processors, and many other automated servants that enable us to be inactive. Sixty percent of American adults are not regularly physically active, and 25% are not active at all.[8] *Find Your Gypsy* suggests ways to get more exercise into your daily life. Fun and exercise don't have to be mutually exclusive. In fact, they shouldn't be if you are looking for a long-term solution that becomes a regular part of your life.

The good news is that making changes *will* make a difference. Bill got the wake up call when he found out he was prediabetic.

He decided it was time to change his diet and lifestyle. He hired some help at work and learned to delegate. He scheduled swimming into his calendar, just as he did his important client meetings. He learned to make healthy choices while eating out. Instead of reaching for a drink as soon as he got home, he made it a tradition to take a short walk with his wife and kids before dinner. Although it was hard to find more time for sleep, even with the diet and other lifestyle changes, Bill noticed he had more energy. It took two years to reverse his prediabetes, but he did it. He also lost that extra 40 pounds and his cholesterol numbers returned to the normal range.

Bill's story brings up an important point about self-medicating. Bill's drug of choice was alcohol, but many others turn to prescription drugs. The rate of antidepressant use in the U.S. increased nearly 400% from 1988-1994 as compared to 2005-2008. Over 10% of Americans take an antidepressant.[9] I've seen this in my own practice, with many clients taking Lexapro, Zoloft, or Prozac to make themselves feel better. Because of the prevalent use of prescription medication in this country, an entire chapter is devoted to the topic. *Just Say Maybe* shows how deadly prescription medications can be. They have a time and a place, but should be used mindfully. You may think you are taking them to make yourself feel better, when they are, in fact, making you sicker.

Eating well, exercising more, sleeping enough, and being mindful of prescription drug use are all ways to nourish your body, and will be further explored in the following chapters. Additional topics include using natural products, being your own health expert, and listening to your body.

Read on to learn about changes you can make in your Body to promote your overall health.

13

Living in the 80s

I've studied nutrition. I know what's good for me to eat and what's not good for me to eat. However, this doesn't mean that I'm perfect all of the time. I'm a big advocate of the 80/20 rule. I try to eat healthy 80% of the time. When I am in the 20% and eating unhealthier foods, I try to be mindful of what I eat so that I savor every bite.

Eating healthy 100% of the time is not realistic and can be unhealthy. Dr. Steven Bratman coined the term orthorexia nervosa, the unhealthy obsession with eating healthy food. If we strive for perfection, we may feel like we have failed whenever we eat unhealthy food. This can cause stress—and, as we know from Part One of this book, the Mind quadrant, stress is not good for our health. In addition, part of health is pleasure. If we deprive ourselves of our favorite foods or feel we cannot (or should not) share a celebration meal with our friends and family because of the food being served, it affects our health. Stressing about eating is counterproductive to our health.

Although most of the time I live in the over 80% zone of eating healthy, there are times when I get on a roll of mindless or unhealthy eating. Whenever I find myself drifting south of 80, I try one or more of the eight tips highlighted below:

1. **Throw it out.** Sometimes you need to help yourself and throw out unhealthy food. I'm giving you permission. It may seem like a waste of money, but it's better than eating it and compromising your health. The key is to be in tune

with your current state of willpower. If you can have a treat in your house and eat small portions every so often, you are in a high willpower state. If, on the other hand, you find yourself finishing the full box of cookies or the entire gallon of ice cream you recently bought, you are in a low willpower state. Be honest with yourself. Our moments of strength and weakness come and go depending on what else is going on in our lives. The best way you can help yourself in times of weakness is to remove the temptation. My clients have said that giving themselves permission to throw out the tempting food has been liberating.

2. **Reduce portion size.** Think about this quote from Orson Welles the next time you serve yourself a plate of food: *"My doctor told me to stop having intimate dinners for four. Unless there are three other people."* Americans on average consume 92% of what is put on our plate, so it's important to pay attention to how much we are serving ourselves. A great way to eat less is to use smaller serving plates. A two inch difference in plate diameter—from 12" to 10"—results in 22% fewer calories being served. This could result in a weight loss of approximately 18 pounds per year for an average adult.[10]

3. **Wait before having seconds.** If you are still hungry, allow 15 to 20 minutes before reaching for seconds. It takes this long for the fullness in your stomach to reach your brain, which is why you can reach the point of being stuffed when you eat a second portion quickly after your first serving. By the time it registers in your brain that you are full, you have eaten well beyond that point. Giving yourself time before you go back for seconds may be just enough time to realize you don't really want any more.

4. **Keep it simple.** I like to eat healthy but I don't like to cook. As a result, my meals are very simple. I don't cook with a lot of sauce, cheese, or butter (though butter *is* preferable to margarine because it doesn't contain trans fats). Eating healthy doesn't have to mean spending a lot of time on preparing the food. Sometimes keeping it simple can be the easiest way to eat healthy.

5. **Eat more veggies.** It is probably safe to say that vegetables are the least controversial food group. Fill up at least half of your plate with vegetables. A creative way to work them into your diet for picky adults and children is to grind them up in a food processor and add them to soups, sauces, or shakes.

6. **Eat mindfully.** Rather than eating in front of the TV, at your desk, or in your car, take time to enjoy your meal. A great way to slow it down is to eat with your non-dominant hand or with chopsticks. You can also try putting down your fork in between bites. Take the time to chew your food which will help slow down the meal process and aid your digestion. Think about what you are eating and the process it went through to get to your plate. Experience the food from your five senses—taste, touch, sound, smell, and sight. Does the food taste bitter, sweet, sour, or salty? Is the texture smooth or crunchy? When you pay attention to the sensation of eating a meal and think about what you are eating, you are more likely to want to make healthy choices.

7. **Dine out with care.** Opt for eating at home more often than not since making healthy choices while dining out can be a challenge. When you do eat out, here are a few tips that can help. Order salad dressing and sauces on the side

so that you can control how much goes on your meal. Better yet, use lemon or vinegar to top your salads. Split a meal or take some home since portion sizes are typically quite large in restaurants. Substitute salad or fruit for fries. Don't be shy about asking for a meal exactly how you want it. Even if the waiter rolls his eyes because you've made three changes and two substitutions to your meal, be proud. You're doing it for your health.

8. **Ask yourself why.** If you find yourself regularly reaching for unhealthy food, ask yourself why you are doing it. Are you doing it for comfort? For many of us, eating is tied to emotion. Sometimes we eat because we are bored, anxious, depressed, or angry. Eating unhealthy food makes us temporarily feel better (or at least we think it will). It is helpful to understand what you are really looking for in the bag of potato chips or box of cookies. Ask yourself, "Why am I reaching for this food and what will it really take to satisfy this need?" For example, if you are angry with someone, you may reach for ice cream instead of confronting the situation.

Taking a moment before you eat may help to pinpoint exactly what is going on with your emotions. Try journaling, writing a letter (that doesn't need to be sent), or talking to a friend about it. Perhaps taking a walk or breathing can keep the emotional eating at bay. If you take a moment to experience your emotions rather than numbing them with food, you can regain control. You will realize that you have a choice as to how you respond to the emotion. It can be either by reaching for food or by doing something that will better satisfy what you really need.

If you are in a period where your healthy eating is below the 80% mark, don't beat yourself up about it. There are good days (weeks) and bad ones. Try again tomorrow. During these times, try a few of the tips mentioned above to see if you can get your eating pattern back up to a higher percentage of the healthy range. And remember, it's okay (even healthy) to be in the 20%—as long as you are there for the right reasons and enjoying it fully (without guilt).

Where are you on the 80/20 scale? If you are south of 80, which of the ideas above might work for you to get back to a higher range? I know you can do it. I'm right there with you.

14

Find Your Gypsy

When you think of the word "exercise," what comes to mind? Does it come with a sense of obligation and a limited view of what qualifies? If you aren't hitting the treadmill or pumping weights a certain number of times per week, do you feel like an exercise failure? When working out isn't something you look forward to doing, the odds of your keeping up with it are greatly reduced. It is important to be creative and think outside the box.

How about this instead…You are riding on your cruiser bike whose name is Gypsy. She has red spokes, tassels on her handlebars, painted flowers on the fenders, and a very cute basket. When you ride her, you feel like a kid again. You ride around the neighborhood streets and parks, appreciating the beauty of nature, the kids playing, and the people out walking their dogs. In no time, you realize that 30 minutes have flown by. Aren't you more likely to have success incorporating this form of movement into your day than one that isn't as fun and appealing? It certainly works for me. I look forward to my rides on Gypsy.

There are many different activities that you can consider "exercise." The important thing is to find what is fun for you and make it a part of your daily living. Here are eight ideas to getting more movement in your day.

1. **Change your framework.** A standard theme I have found with my clients is the guilt that comes with the "should" of exercising. Leave behind the "should" and find your "want." Think of "exercise" as movement that brings you joy. Traditional types of exercise like hiking, biking, running,

swimming, kayaking, dancing, skiing, and tennis can be incorporated into your daily life if you focus more on the fun and less on the result. After training for marathons for a few years, running started to feel more like an obligation to me. I decided to leave the heart rate monitor, distance watch, and speed expectations at home. As a result, I found joy in my running again.

2. **Think creatively.** My dad doesn't like to go to the gym, but he does like to walk his neighborhood. He lives in the desert, so in the summer it's too hot to walk outside. During the warmer months, he gets creative. He walks inside an air-conditioned mall. This also works well for those who live in cold temperature locations during the winter months. If it's not mall walking, maybe it's hula hooping? It's a great abdominal workout and it's fun too. Jumping rope is good cardio and reminds us of our childhood days. My husband has recently taken up jumping on a pogo stick. He gets a good workout and he brings joy to the neighborhood. How can you not laugh seeing a grown man bouncing down the street on a pogo stick? How about a game of hopscotch, Frisbee, or basketball? Or turning on the stereo and dancing around to your favorite music? The point is, be creative and playful. If it gets you moving, it counts as exercise. It will lower your stress and put a smile on your face.

3. **Make the gym fun.** Some people like the gym. If you are one of them, that's great. You don't need to be creative like the rest of us to get exercise into your life. Keep it up! For those of us who need a little nudge to get to the gym, think about how to make it more enticing. Can you go at a certain time to watch a show you like? Download some music that is reserved only for your gym workouts? Meet a friend? Try

a new class? If you are bored with your typical gym class, try belly dancing or boxing instead. It will be fun and a great workout to boot. I tried Zumba recently and couldn't stop laughing at how ridiculous I looked, but I got a good workout.

4. **Talk and walk.** Instead of meeting your friends for coffee or lunch, meet them for a walk. You save money and you get some exercise. This is my mom's favorite form of exercise. She says that she spends so much time gabbing that she forgets her legs are doing a lot of walking.

5. **Do it with someone.** It is easier to cancel out on yourself than on someone else. Having support from others can get you through on the challenging days. Sign up for a tennis class, join a hiking group, or participate in one of the many charity organizations that walk and run various distance races. Offer to start a walking group at your doctor's office, children's school, or religious community. Check out Meetup.com for local groups. It doesn't matter what it is, just do it with someone.

6. **Count your steps.** Wearing a pedometer is a great motivator. Set a goal of at least 7,000 steps a day (10,000 is ideal). Make it a family activity and see who can get the most steps in a week. Walking is a great way to stay healthy. Be prepared by keeping comfortable shoes in your car so that you can go for a walk any time you find yourself with a free moment.

7. **Crunch at work.** We spend so much of our time at work that it is beneficial to find ways to move while on the job. I recently got a treadmill desk. This is a stand-up desk that fits over a treadmill. It may seem like it would be hard to

get work done while walking, but it's not because it is designed to go slow. I am able to talk on the phone and work on the computer while walking. The miles add up. In two weeks, I have spent 30 of my working hours walking. Typically I would have been sitting for those hours. Instead, I walked 42 miles. I know other people who work while pedaling on their stationary bike. If these aren't feasible options, you can make it as simple as delivering documents in person rather than using interoffice mail or walking to a different floor to use the restroom. My client, Christie, says that she and her colleagues have started doing mini group workouts every hour. They take a few minutes at the top of each hour to do exercises like marching in place, chair crunches, and squats. She says, "It's like a shot of espresso."

8. **Keep moving.** Try to move throughout the day rather than think of "exercise" as something you do at a certain time and then are done. For example, take the stairs instead of the elevator, park in a far spot at the grocery store, or do your own gardening. At home, try walking around when you are on the phone or stretching while watching television. Even cleaning your house counts as movement.

Research shows that a lack of exercise increases risk of diseases such as cancer, diabetes, osteoporosis, and heart disease. It also shows that a commitment to exercise can prevent disease. Whatever way you look at it, exercise is good for your health! It enhances your mood, improves your energy, helps you sleep better, boosts your immune system, lowers your blood pressure, increases your metabolism, helps you maintain a healthy weight, and so much more.

I love my time on Gypsy and look forward to getting out for a ride every chance I get. What is your Gypsy?

15

From A's to Zzzzs

When I was a kid, I remember learning about Ponce de Leon, a Spanish explorer in the 16th century, searching for the fountain of youth. Perhaps if he had spent more time sleeping and less time searching, he would have found it. The fountain of youth is sleep!

We are a society that is driven to perfection. We need to get an "A" in all areas of our lives—being a parent, spouse, worker, friend, child, and so on. Focusing on getting "A's" often means getting fewer Zzzzs. The demands on our time are starting so early these days. Look at how busy kids are with all of their in-school and after-school activities. Life is a lot more frenetic than it used to be. We are averaging one to two hours less sleep a night today than our grandparents. In fact, 43% of adults say that they are so sleepy during the day that it interferes with their daily activity and 60% of children under the age of 18 say they are tired during the school day (with 15% admitting they fall asleep in class).[11]

Sleep is highly underrated. It is not something that is "nice to have;" it is essential for our health. In fact, lack of sleep impacts motor skills so severely that driving while sleep deprived is comparable to drunk driving. Sleepy drivers cause at least 100,000 car accidents in the U.S. each year.[12] Not getting enough sleep also weakens our immune system, which puts us at greater risk of disease and infection. And, it increases stress, anxiety, and depression. It has also been linked to weight gain.

Sleep is a natural antidote to the damage done to our bodies during the course of the day. During sleep, our bodies replenish the immune system, eliminate free radicals, ward off heart disease, and alleviate our mood imbalances. Melatonin, a naturally occurring sleep-regulating hormone (triggered when the lights go out), has been linked to lower cancer risk. When you get a good night's sleep, your body produces more melatonin. Clearly, it's time to start taking sleep seriously.

Are you and your children getting enough sleep? If you fall asleep as soon as you get into bed at night, have difficulty waking up in the morning, are moody and irritable, or fall asleep at work or in class, you may be sleep deprived. Generally, 8 hours of sleep is the norm, though the range people need varies from 6 to 10 hours. If you suffer from a sleep disorder, including insomnia, excessive drowsiness, sleep apnea, and restless movement during sleep, you are not alone. About 70 million Americans also suffer from this condition.[13]

There are many factors that can affect your sleep including stress, hormonal changes, excessive caffeine, little or no exercise, shift work, and alcohol consumption. Many people turn to prescription drugs to help them sleep. Instead, try these 10 natural ways for getting a good night's sleep:

1. **Go dark and quiet.** Sleep in complete darkness and silence. If you don't have a dark room, wear an eye mask. For silence, use earplugs.

2. **Stop the caffeine.** Don't drink caffeinated beverages after lunch. My client, Karen, had major sleeping issues, waking every night around three in the morning and not being able to go back to sleep. As soon as she stopped drinking coffee in the morning and energy drinks throughout the day, she slept through the night.

3. **Eat a bedtime snack.** Try eating a snack before bed that is a complex carbohydrate paired with a protein, such as apples with almond butter, carrots with hummus, or a cup of oatmeal with milk. Of course, it needs to be a healthy snack in a small portion size and factored in to your total daily food intake. Having a nighttime snack could be beneficial for those who have trouble with blood sugar regulation or sleeping throughout the night.

4. **Relax and breathe.** Learn and practice a relaxation technique to do before bedtime, such as breathing exercises, gentle yoga, or meditation. Listening to music, taking a bath, or drinking a hot cup of herbal tea can help too. For more information on meditationg and breathing, see *Meditation with Hollywood* and *Rise and Fall* in Part One, the Mind quadrant.

5. **Write it out.** Keep a journal and write in it before you go to sleep. How many of us lie in bed with our minds going a mile a minute? Write your thoughts down before bed to get them out of your head. Try visually thinking about taking your thoughts out of your head and putting them into a box that sits at the far corner of the room. Take comfort knowing that the box will be there in the morning for you to pick up where you left off, if you so choose. For the nighttime hours, free your mind. Use whatever method works for you. The idea is to quiet the mental chatter in your head by getting your thoughts out before you try to sleep.

6. **Watch the liquids.** Avoid drinking too many fluids within two hours of going to bed to minimize trips to the bathroom.

7. **Exercise early.** Exercising regularly is great for getting a good night's sleep. Try not to do it too close to bedtime or you may have trouble falling asleep because your body is still pumped up with adrenaline from your workout.

8. **Create bedroom bliss.** Make your bedroom a place for sleeping—not for watching TV, eating, or working. This works for several of my clients, but I must confess that my nightly ritual of watching television in bed right before I sleep (while eating my nighttime snack) is relaxing. It's all about doing what works best for you and creating your own bedroom bliss.

9. **Stop smoking.** Nicotine is a stimulant. Of course, not smoking will bring you many health benefits in addition to better sleep.

10. **Don't drink and sleep.** Alcohol may help put you to sleep faster, but your sleep will be disrupted. If you are having trouble sleeping, try limiting your alcohol consumption.

In today's busy world, we have a lot of demands on our time. Don't sacrifice your sleep time to get it all done. In the long run, it will end up reducing your productivity and compromising your health.

Ponce de Leon never found the fountain, but you can. Just get more Zzzzzs. What steps will you take to get a better night's sleep?

16

Keeping It Real

"I'm not a fake human, so why am I feeding myself fake food?" My client, Leslie, asked herself this question after I showed her the ingredients in the meal replacement bars she ate daily. She thought these bars were healthy. She chose them because they were gluten-free and were lower in calories and fat than some of the other bars.

Leslie realized that when she ate the bar, she wasn't eating real food. The ingredient list started off with soy protein isolate, followed with a few types of sugar like evaporated cane juice and brown rice syrup, and ended with a long list of items we couldn't pronounce. I suggested opting instead for real food that was just as convenient, like a nut and dried fruit mix.

When you are shopping the aisles of a grocery store, how do you choose what you put in your cart? Is it the promise on the front of the label that the product is fat-free, gluten-free, or sugar-free? Do you look at the back of the packaging to see how many calories or grams of carbohydrates are in it? The single most important area on packaged goods labeling is actually the ingredient list. This is where you can determine whether the food is real or fake.

Simply looking at the number of calories or fat grams doesn't tell the whole story of whether the item is what Michael Pollan, author of *In Defense of Food* and *Food Rules*, calls an "edible food-like substance." These foods are highly processed and are designed by food scientists. They consist mostly of ingredients derived from corn and soy along with some chemical additives. There are 17,000 new products that show up in our supermarkets each year that are faux foods.

The general rule of thumb is that less is more when it comes to ingredients. A healthier choice for breakfast instead of cereal is steel-cut oatmeal or eggs. The ingredient list for eggs is "egg" and the ingredient list for oatmeal is "oats." When you pick up a product with a long and complicated ingredient list, let it be a red flag that you are holding a faux food item. Ingredients that you cannot pronounce are likely manufactured. If the package has ingredients like diglycerides, cellulose, xanthan gum, or ammonium sulfate, leave it behind. Most of these food science ingredients are put in the product to extend shelf life and to encourage you to eat more (via our propensity for sweet, fat, and salt).

No-fat foods may look great on the stats, but when you look at the ingredients, you can see that all of the nutrients and wholeness of the food have been stripped to make the nutrition facts look good. There is a perception that fat can cause fat, but we have actually gotten fatter as a nation living on no-fat and low-fat foods. These no-fat foods typically contain more sugar and are not as satisfying as their full fat counterparts (which means we eat more of it).

Eating fat does not cause fat. In fact, recent studies confirm that healthy fat consumption actually promotes sustainable weight loss and keeps the cells in our body healthy.[14] You just need to be eating the right fat. Healthy fats include avocados, nuts, seeds, almond butter, olive oil, coconut oil, and eggs.

It wouldn't be a complete discussion about real food without mentioning GMOs (genetically modified organisms). Most GMOs are designed to produce their own insecticide to fight bugs or to withstand increasing dosages of weed killer. While this is fascinating from a science standpoint, it is disturbing from a health standpoint.

Genetically modified foods are becoming increasingly prevalent in this country. Nearly 80% of processed foods in the U.S. have GMOs.[15]

The top nine genetically engineered food crops are corn, soy, canola, cotton, papaya, alfalfa, sugar beets, zucchini, and yellow summer squash. When reading labels, it may not always be obvious if the product contains GMOs since the ingredients listed—such as xanthan gum, sucrose, maltodextrins, citric acid, and high fructose corn syrup—could have been derived from these crops. Milk, meat, and eggs can also contain GMOs from the food that the animals eat.

Because countries like Canada, the United Kingdom, New Zealand, and all 27 countries in Europe do not allow things like artificial growth hormones, food dyes derived from petrochemicals, and genetically engineered ingredients into their food supplies, global companies must make a different version to compete in the marketplace abroad. Below is a look at the difference between U.S. and U.K. Kraft Mac & Cheese.

U.S. Version of Kraft Mac & Cheese:
Enriched Macaroni Product (Wheat Flour, Niacin, Ferrous Sulfate [Iron], Thiamin Mononitrate [Vitamin B1], Riboflavin [Vitamin B2], Folic Acid), Cheese Sauce Mix (Whey, Modified Food Starch, Whey Protein Concentrate, Cheddar Cheese [Milk, Cheese Culture, Salt, Enzymes], Salt, Calcium Carbonate, Potassium Chloride, Contains Less Than 2% of Parmesan Cheese [Part-Skim Milk, Cheese Culture, Salt, Enzymes, Dried Buttermilk, Sodium Tripolyphosphate, Blue Cheese [Milk, Cheese Culture, Salt, Enzymes], Sodium Phosphate, Medium Chain Triglycerides, Cream, Citric Acid, Lactic Acid, Enzymes, Yellow 5, Yellow 6).

U.K. Version of Kraft Mac & Cheese:
Macaroni (Durum Wheat Semolina), Cheese (10%), Whey Powder (from milk), Lactose, Salt, Emulsifying Salts (E339, E341), Colours (Paprika Extract, Beta-Carotene)

The U.K. version has no dyes and fewer (better) ingredients. Instead of using Yellow 5 and 6 to get the desired color, they use natural ingredients like paprika extract and beta-carotene. Why are we allowing this to happen in our country?

As voters, we should encourage the government to follow suit like the other countries. (California tried to lead the way with Prop 37 in 2012, seeking mandatory labeling of genetically modified foods, but it was voted down.) As consumers, we should demand the healthier version of food products. As eaters, we should opt for whole foods that do not contain hormones or pesticides, and avoid foods that have been genetically modified.

Certified organic foods are not allowed to contain genetically engineered ingredients, so buying organic ensures you avoid GMOs. Some products have "GMO-free" listed on their packaging, but there are currently no government regulations on such labeling. The Non-GMO Project can provide you with more information about buying foods free of GMOs.

Remember that when it comes to making healthy food choices, less is more. Keep it simple and stick to whole foods. With this strategy, you can't go wrong. As Pollan says, *"If it came from a plant, eat it; if it was made in a plant, don't."* It doesn't get much clearer than that.

What edible foodlike substances posing as real food are lurking in your cupboards?

17

Au Natural

Sandra wakes up in the morning and fixes herself an egg scramble with spinach and onions. She even squeezes some fresh oranges for juice to go along with it. Sandra feels great about how much care she put into her food choice this morning, opting for real food. She then gets ready for the day, washing her face, brushing her teeth, shampooing her hair, putting lotion on her body, and applying makeup.

We often take great care in what we put in our bodies (food), but don't think twice about what we put on our bodies (products). Our skin is highly permeable. It is often quoted that up to sixty percent of the product we put on our skin is absorbed into our body. Since skin is our largest organ, we are putting a lot of product on our skin and thus into our bloodstream.

Think about how many personal care products you are using in a day. Is it five? Ten? On average, we use nine personal care products per day, resulting in 126 unique ingredients on our skin daily.[16] Food has the benefit of passing through the liver for some detoxification, but what we put on our skin goes straight into our bloodstream without this filtering.

It's hard to believe, but the government does not require any testing or health studies for personal care products before they go to market. There is no requirement that companies test products for safety before they reach the store shelves. There is a self-policing safety panel, the Cosmetics Ingredients Review, but they have not reviewed more than half of the thousands of ingredients companies use in cosmetics.

When you are using body wash, shampoo, lotion, toothpaste, and makeup, you could be putting toxins into your body. These exposures can result in skin irritations, headaches, dizziness, vomiting, and more. They can also disrupt your endocrine, immune, reproductive, respiratory, and nervous systems. Below is a look at some of the top synthetic chemicals to avoid commonly found in beauty products, along with their negative health consequences.[17]

- **Parabens.** Parabens extend the shelf life of products. They include ethyl, methyl, butyl, or propyl in the prefix. They are found in lotions, shaving cream, makeup, and shower products. The FDA currently considers parabens safe, but many researchers fear they are toxic. They can cause allergic reactions and skin rashes, and have been found in some breast cancer tumors. Research on parabens and cancer is inconclusive, but products without them are likely to be safer.

- **Fragrance.** Fragrance gives a product its pleasant smell. However, the term "fragrance" can indicate the presence of up to 4,000 separate ingredients. Many are toxic or carcinogenic. They can affect the central nervous system, causing depression, hyperactivity, and irritability. Symptoms include headaches, dizziness, skin irritations, allergic rashes, violent coughing, and vomiting.

- **Phthalates.** Phthalates are found in some nail polishes, hair sprays, and are commonly hidden under the term "fragrance." Phthalates are also found in toys, plastic wrap, cleaning sprays, and more. Phthalates are endocrine-disruptors linked to lower testosterone levels, reduced female fertility, a worsening of allergy and asthma symptoms, and behavior changes.

- **Sodium Lauryl Sulfate (SLS).** SLS is used in most products that foam, including cleansers, shampoos, shower gels, and toothpaste. It is also used in garage floor cleaners, engine degreasers, and car wash soaps. It causes eye irritations, skin rashes, hair loss, and other allergic reactions.

- **Propylene Glycol.** This substance retains moisture and is often found in skin moisturizers and deodorants. It was originally developed as an anti-freeze and is the major ingredient in brake and hydraulic fluid. It is a skin irritant that causes allergic reactions and acne. It may also cause liver and kidney problems.

- **Other Products.** Other products to avoid include **Petrolatum** (also listed as **Mineral Oil** or **Paraffin**), **Triclosan**, **Polyethylene Glycol** (PEG), and **Synthetic Colors** (FD&C, D&C).

Here are six ideas for reducing your toxic exposure:

1. **Support the right companies.** Personal care products can be made with healthier ingredients. Opt for products that are based on plant oils instead of petrochemicals, colors derived from natural minerals such as titanium dioxide, fragrances from essential oils, and natural preservatives such as vitamins C and E or grapefruit seed extract. There may be a non-toxic shampoo that you like just as much as the one you are using, so why not choose that one?

2. **Read the ingredients.** It is important to read the label and

buy products with the fewest ingredients. Don't rely on the marketing label to tell you if the product is natural. Review the list and decide for yourself. If you don't know what the ingredient is, it's probably a manufactured chemical.

3. **Use fewer products.** Be mindful when using your personal care products and see what you can use less often or cut out entirely. For example, when my skin isn't dry, I don't use lotion. Don't use products merely because they are part of a routine or are socially expected.

4. **Know your resources.** Go online and check out Environmental Working Group's Skin Deep Cosmetic Safety Database or GoodGuide. Type in your product to find its toxicity rating. If you want a comprehensive list of toxic ingredients, buy *Toxic Beauty* by Samuel Epstein and Randall Fitzgerald. They have a tear-out sheet with a list of over 200 toxic ingredients, and they identify whether the ingredient is an allergen, carcinogen, hormone disrupter, penetration enhancer, formaldehyde releaser, or neurotoxin.

5. **Check the expiration.** Look for products with expiration dates. Compounds may change and cause a new reaction or have limited effectiveness. Keep in mind that natural products are more likely to expire if preservatives aren't used.

6. **Give it the spoon test.** If you wouldn't put it on a spoon and eat it, think twice about putting it on your skin or hair.

Are there any products in your bathroom cabinet or vanity that you are willing to trade in for an "au natural" version?

18

Just Say Maybe

Last year my mom was rushed to the emergency room right after taking a drug for a sinus infection. She was lightheaded, shaking, and short of breath. Her hands and feet were freezing. Her doctor said that it was unlikely the reaction was from the medication, despite the fact that the symptoms happened immediately upon taking the first pill. After doing some research, I found many others who had experienced the same side effects after taking that particular drug.

Despite their best intentions, doctors, the FDA, and pharmaceutical companies do not have all the answers. We need to watch out for our own best interests by being empowered health consumers and taking medications mindfully—prescription drugs as well as over-the-counter medicines.

My mom is not alone. Each year, an estimated two million Americans are hospitalized from adverse reactions to prescription medication and over 100,000 Americans actually die from these drugs. The average patient takes more than 12 prescription medications each year. We are also drugging our children, which is frightening. In recent years, prescription spending rose faster for children than for any other group.[18] Teenage prescription drug abuse is on the rise as well. One in four teens has misused or abused a prescription drug at least once in their lifetime.[19]

We tend to accept whatever prescription our doctor gives us, without doing our own research on whether it is right for us to take. There are numerous, serious side effects to many medications. There are also complications with certain medications when taken in conjunction with other prescription drugs. We often do not realize that we feel sick *because* of the drugs we are taking. In addition, these drugs often do not heal or cure. They simply mask our symptoms without getting to the root of the problem. For example, taking blood pressure medication only lowers your blood pressure while you are on the medication. It does not treat the underlying cause. You will need to be on it for life *unless* you make changes to your diet and lifestyle to bring your blood pressure down naturally.

We have a false sense of security that if a drug is approved, it must be safe. There have been many drugs removed from the market after they were shown to be fatal. Vioxx, a drug by Merck, was approved by the FDA in 1999. It was marketed as a nonsteroidal anti-inflammatory drug used to treat osteoarthritis and acute pain conditions. Internal studies at Merck showed that Vioxx did not relieve pain any better than the far cheaper over-the-counter ibuprofen options, but Merck still launched and marketed the drug. Within a year after its release, the FDA noted problems with the drug's side effects, notably heart attacks, cardiac deaths, and strokes, and required Merck to add a warning label. Merck had already identified these issues with the drug—two years before its release.

Vioxx remained on the market, with Merck spending 160 million dollars on advertising in one year. (It is interesting to note that the U.S. is one of only two countries—the other being New Zealand—that allows direct-to-consumer advertising, such as television and prints ads, for pharmaceutical drugs.) Vioxx was finally pulled in 2004 after substantial litigation and media attention. Merck made $2.5 billion in sales revenue during its five years on the market. The gains came at a steep price; worldwide, 100,000 people died from the drug.[20] Unfortunately, Vioxx is not an isolated example.

I mention Vioxx to underscore the point that just because a drug is on the market does not mean it is safe. Take medications with awareness and only as needed. Do the research. Find out about the side effects and pay attention while you are taking the drug to see if you are experiencing any of them. If you are, contact your doctor immediately. Find out if the medication can interfere with any other medications you are taking or can aggravate another health condition you might have.

This is not to say that all prescription drugs are inherently bad. There may be a time and place for them. In fact, in some cases, it may be the most effective solution. For example, medications for serious asthma attacks and severe allergic reactions can be real life-savers.

AskAPatient.com, operated by Consumer Health Resource Group, is a great resource for finding out about side effects that other people have experienced from over 4,000 FDA approved prescription drugs. It is important to realize that even though the chemistry of the drug may be well understood, the chemistry of how it interacts within our bodies varies by individual. Because we each have our own biochemical individuality, our reactions to drugs can differ. Just because a certain medication worked without side effects for a friend or family member, does not mean it will work the same way for you.

Before reaching for the medications, try exploring natural ways to take care of health concerns—for you, your family, and even your pets. Natural remedies can be just as effective without the side effects. For example, exercise in combination with weight loss can reduce the odds of developing diabetes by 58%, nearly double the rate of success of diabetes medication (31%).[21] There are numerous ideas throughout this book offering natural ways to promote health to reduce the need to turn to prescription drugs.

Your body is an amazing self-healer. Give it the time it needs without reaching for the antibiotics if you feel a sniffle coming on. Think twice about putting potentially harmful pills into your body unless you absolutely have to. Research how your condition can be treated naturally and look into all drugs before consuming.

Next time you are given a prescription, will you "just say maybe"?

19

The Trendy Diet

Are you on the trendy diet? Have you been riding the roller coaster of the latest nutrition fads fueled by the media? This phenomenon has been going on for over 150 years.

If you were alive in the 1860s, being on the trendy diet would mean you *wouldn't* be eating carbs. If you were alive in the 1980s, you *would* be eating carbs. And, if you were alive in the early 2000s, you *wouldn't* be eating them again. Carbs are bad, carbs are good, and carbs are bad. The same fate was shared by fat. It was good, then it was bad, and now it is good again (the good fats). Soy was a nutrition darling for a while and then it got blacklisted. Eggs have been on and off the trendy diet too. In the current day, wheat seems to be the latest nutrition enemy.

Gary Taubes in *Good Calories, Bad Calories* gives a detailed historical account of the diet phenomenon, underscoring the fickleness of it all. The first popular diet craze came in 1863 when William Banting, an obese man who tried a diet mostly of protein while avoiding sugar and starch foods, wrote about how he lost 50 pounds. This led to the first diet frenzy—carbs are bad, fat is good.

Carbs lasted as the enemy for over a century. And then, in the mid 1980s, the tide began to change. At this point, carbs became heart-healthy food. We were told that it was now the butter rather than the bread that was the enemy. In the 1980s, the American Heart Association identified dietary fat as a probable cause of heart disease and advocated low-fat diets as a means of prevention.

Low-fat and no-fat foods lined the shelves of supermarkets, most of them stripped of their nutrients and with added sugars to make them taste good.

The tide turned again. In the early 2000s, low-carb diets, such as the Atkins diet, became widely popular. These diets returned us to the trend that fat is good, (simple) carbs are bad.

In another nutritional controversy, we've also been fickle about soy. For a while, soy was the end-all, be-all—especially as a benefit for breast cancer prevention. People were loading up on tofu and edamame. A few years later, we were cautioned that too much soy could, in fact, be harmful. Women concerned about breast cancer were told to limit their soy intake.

The changing tide of nutrition is the reality of our culture. New "research" comes to light, suggesting new ideas which become the latest craze. Product companies make their money jumping on the latest bandwagon and fueling the diet fad frenzy.

The latest enemy appears to be wheat. Supermarket shelves are now lined with gluten-free foods. Restaurants are promoting their wheat-free items. It is important to remember that just because a food is "gluten-free" does not mean it is a healthy food (like we saw with the no-fat craze). Many gluten-free products are made of refined carbs and added fats. They also typically lack key nutrients and fiber that are found in their fortified wheat counterparts.

Why is wheat getting a bad rap? Wheat in the U.S. tends to be overly processed and stripped of its nutrients. Some believe it is inflammatory because we are not built to digest gluten, the protein found in wheat. Wheat today has more gluten in it than it did in the past so this may be why we are seeing an increase in reactions to gluten.

Some people certainly should not be eating products containing gluten. Others are scared to. If you have been diagnosed with celiac disease, you should be avoiding all grains that include gluten such as wheat, barley, rye, spelt, and faro. Celiac disease, an autoimmune disease in which a person can't tolerate gluten, can be diagnosed with genetic testing. Even if you do not have the celiac gene, you may still be sensitive to gluten.

The best way to know if you are sensitive to gluten or any other type of food is to avoid eating it for a few weeks and see if you feel better. Then try reintroducing the food into your diet and note how you feel right after eating it and for several days after. Food sensitivities can show up as long as 72 hours later. Some of the symptoms you may experience are gastrointestinal distress, skin irritations, difficulty breathing during exercise, fatigue, and headaches. The top allergenic foods include dairy, wheat, nuts, soy, shellfish, and eggs.

Do you tend to follow the trendy diet? If so, try the 12 healthy eating tips discussed in *Fad-Free Eating* that stand the test of time.

Will you stay off the trendy diet and do your own research so that *you* can make the decision of what food is best for you?

20
Follow Yourself

You are your own best advocate of your health. You are the one most motivated to help yourself. The government, your doctors, the pharmaceutical companies, your friends, and your family all may have the best intentions for you, but you are the one that knows the most about what is best for you.

My neighbor had breast cancer a couple of years ago and had chemotherapy as treatment. She ended up in the hospital from a severe reaction to it. Recently, her doctors recommended chemotherapy again for a new cancer. She didn't want to do it. Her gut told her it wasn't right for her, but her doctor and husband encouraged her. She listened to them and did it. She ended up in the hospital again, this time with a heart attack. Even while she was in the hospital from the heart attack, her husband told her she should still continue with the chemotherapy. She knew, as she had known before, that chemotherapy was not the right course of treatment for her. She is now following her instinct and not doing any additional chemotherapy treatments. She is trying other conventional and some alternative treatments that feel right for her and her body.

This is not about the pros and cons of chemotherapy; this is about trusting yourself to know what is best for you. My neighbor knew that chemotherapy was not right for her, but she let herself get talked into it with near fatal consequences. My sister had Stage 3 breast cancer and is 15 years cancer-free. She had very aggressive chemotherapy treatments and would be the first to tell you that these treatments saved her life.

There is not one right solution for everyone. We are all different in our biochemical makeup and, as a result, we will have varying reactions to treatments. Do what is right for you. Remember that you are the expert on your own health. You know what is best for your body. Trust yourself. See your doctors as partners in your health care. Listen to what they have to say and decide for yourself if it is right for you.

Doctors and hospitals are not without error. Every year in the U.S., there are hundreds of thousands of deaths induced inadvertently by a physician, surgeon, medical treatment, or diagnostic procedure. The estimate of these annual deaths ranges from 250,000 to 800,000, depending on which categories are included.[22] The high end includes deaths by infection, medical error, adverse drug reactions, bedsores, malnutrition, surgery-related, and unnecessary procedures. Whether we choose the low-end or high-end number, these deaths are one of the leading causes of deaths in the U.S. There is no question that the medical system saves lives, but it is important to be an empowered, educated, and active health consumer.

My client, Dan, went to a doctor who wanted him to sign a document that said he would do exactly what the doctor told him to do. If he did not sign the document and adhere to the recommendations, the doctor would no longer treat my client. Dan sought treatment elsewhere.

If your doctor does not make time for you or listen to you, or will only treat you if you follow the prescribed recommendations, find another doctor. Do your own research, ask questions, and talk to others. As the old adage goes, *"Listen to everyone. Follow no one."* Or better yet, *"Listen to everyone. Follow yourself."* Demand the care you deserve and don't settle for anything less.

Are you ready to take on the role of expert of your health?

21

Diagnosis: Inadequate Eyelashes

How far will we go for beauty? Apparently, pretty far.

Did you know that Latisse, a product people use to lengthen their eyelashes, is actually a side effect of a drug used to treat a serious medical condition? This beauty product originated from a group of popular medications called topical prostaglandins, drugs used for patients with glaucoma, an eye disease. A side effect of this medication is hypertrichosis, a condition characterized by darkening, thickening, and lengthening of the eyelashes. People who do not have glaucoma are taking a prescription medication for the benefit of its side effect. Say what?

Having thin eyelashes is actually considered a medical condition now. Latisse received FDA approval for the "treatment of inadequate eyelashes." Who determined that thick eyelashes are desirable and beautiful? Hair on other parts of our body is undesirable. Beauty is so subjective, yet people are now taking a prescription medication to have thicker lashes.

I think smile lines and gray hair might be medical conditions too. The injectable wrinkle filler, LaViv, made from your own skin tissue was recently approved by the FDA for the treatment of smile lines. A few years ago, researchers discovered the proteins that cause gray hair, which led to media reports of "an eventual cure" for gray hair.

Medicalization, a process by which nonmedical conditions become defined and treated as medical problems, is not limited to eyelashes, wrinkles, and gray hair. Natural life events like puberty, childbirth, menopause, and aging have also become medicalized. These stages in life are now "conditions" that require drugs and doctors. The media and pharmaceutical companies are creating disease and selling the cure. We are buying it.

Melody Petersen, in *Our Daily Meds*, gives some powerful and disturbing examples of medicalization. One such example is the disease of bad breath. Pharmaceutical company, Warner-Lambert, expanded the market for Listerine mouthwash in the 1920s by creating public anxiety about halitosis, better known as bad breath. Based on a widespread ad campaign that blamed halitosis for job and relationship troubles, Listerine's net earnings increased forty-fold. One of the ads said, "You 5,000,000 women who want to get married: How's your breath today?" Suddenly bad breath was a social ill and medical condition. Promoting the more serious sounding names, halitosis (bad breath) and hypotrichosis (inadequate eyelashes), seems to legitimize the medical treatment of these bodily happenings.

When I was in high school, I went to see a dermatologist. He put me on Accutane, a serious drug with plenty of short-term and long-term side effects. I was a teenager with a few pimples and I was being treated for the medical condition of puberty.

Once we make it out of the woes of puberty, we have to worry about aging. My sister recently found herself taking allergy medication because the hair dye she was using made her scalp itch. She then came to the realization that if she stopped using that particular hair dye, she wouldn't need the allergy medication. Are you being lured into the frenzy too? It's time to stop the madness.

And, it is madness. Americans spent nearly $10 billion on cosmetic procedures in 2011. There were over nine million surgical and nonsurgical cosmetic procedures performed in the U.S. in 2011. [23] Popular surgical procedures include breast augmentation, liposuction, tummy tuck, breast lift, and eyelid surgery. Popular nonsurgical procedures include Botox, laser hair removal, and microdermabrasion.

A recent magazine article started with the headline, "If you can't tone it, tan it!" The article talked about how being tan can help you look skinnier. It made me think about how we define beauty. There used to be a time when being pale was desirable because it meant you weren't working in the fields. Similarly, being heavier was a sign of prosperity and fertility.

I wonder—with all of the plucking, tweezing, waxing, tanning, dyeing, injecting, and medicating—what disease are we trying to cure? Is it the disease of "unattractiveness"? How can we cure a disease when the diagnosis of unattractiveness is subjective and seems to change over time and with geographic boundaries?

I'm not saying we shouldn't do anything in the name of "beauty" because that isn't realistic. We are all products of our socialization. I am saying we should make it a conscious choice instead of being on autopilot. Make your choices thoughtfully and remember that the food we eat, the people we socialize with, the exercise we do, the way we manage stress—all of these things can give us beauty, anti-aging, health, vitality, and so much more.

What beauty regimen can you forgo or alter in the name of health?

22

Body Talk

Jennifer has high blood pressure. One day I had her take her blood pressure. She recorded the number. Right after that, I led her through a guided meditation to relax her. She took her blood pressure again. It was noticeably lower.

Our body talks and what it has to say can be quite insightful. We can learn from it and reprogram our stress response by understanding what tools and techniques work best to relax us. Listening to our body talk and learning from it is called biofeedback. The before and after monitor readings helped Jennifer see the impact that the relaxation exercise had physiologically in her body.

When something stressful happens, you may feel physiological changes in your body like an increase in your heart rate, breathing, sweating, muscle tension, body temperature, or blood pressure. While this response can be helpful in a fight-or-flight moment, as discussed earlier, it is not good if it is experienced chronically. By tuning in to your body's reactions to stress, you can change your response over time. The goal is to be able to initiate this response at the early warning signs of stress.

Although there are clinical forms of biofeedback where you are hooked up to a machine, you can also do it on your own. You can use a blood pressure monitor or a sports watch heart rate monitor. You can also simply take your own pulse or count your breath.

Try it now. Think of something stressful. List out all the things you have to do in a day or think of someone who makes you tense. Take your pulse (or count your breath) by putting your index and middle finger on the inside of your wrist or neck. Count how many times you feel a pulse in a 30 second time frame. Record the number. Now take a few minutes and breathe deeply (Read *Rise and Fall* in Part One). Visualize being somewhere calming and peaceful for you. Breathe in serenity and breathe out stress.

Now take your pulse (or count your breath) again for 30 seconds. Compare the two numbers. Is your pulse (breath) rate lower the second time around while you were in the relaxed state? By doing this exercise, you have learned that you can affect physiological changes in your body—with something as accessible as deep breathing. This is a powerful insight for managing stress.

You can try various relaxation techniques and coping strategies to see what works best for you. Identify which one lowers your pulse rate the most. All of us are unique and will respond differently. Relaxation techniques include muscle relaxation, affirmations, deep breathing, visualizations, meditation, and listening to calming music. Coping strategies include journal writing, art therapy, humor therapy, creative problem solving, resource management, and reframing.

Hearing our body talk helps us to be more in tune with ourselves and empowers us to take control of our health. It moves us from an outside center of control to an inside one. Biofeedback has been shown to be an effective tool for a host of stress-related health issues, including tension and migraine headaches, hypertension, ulcers, insomnia, asthma, tinnitus, ADD, Raynaud's disease, and gastrointestinal disorders. Modern thinking in neuroscience believes that we can even change the neural pathways in our brain by something as simple as practicing gratitude.

Is your body talking to you and are you listening?

23

Fad-Free Eating

There is so much information about how to eat right, with the recommendations changing frequently. As discussed in the chapter *The Trendy Diet*, new studies come to light—and they often contradict the old studies. Below are the top 12 tips for healthy eating that will stand the test of time.

1. **Eat real food.** As previously mentioned, Michael Pollan refers to the 17,000 new products that show up in our super-markets each year as "edible foodlike substances." These foods are highly processed with very few nutrients. Instead, opt for real foods for healthy eating. The best way to find real food is to shop the perimeter of the grocery store, or better yet, go to your local farmers market. Great real food choices include the following:
   - All fruits and vegetables (berries, broccoli, Brussels sprouts, kale, spinach, sweet potatoes, tomatoes)
   - Nuts (almonds, cashews, walnuts)
   - Beans (black, kidney)
   - Eggs (pastured)
   - Organic lean meats (chicken, turkey)
   - Fish with omega-3 fatty acids (salmon, sardines)
   - Whole grains (brown rice, quinoa)

2. **Follow the rainbow.** How do you ensure you are getting all of the vitamins and nutrients you need? You don't have to

know which foods contain vitamin C or beta-carotene. Instead, simply eat a variety of colors. This will ensure you get the nutrients your body needs without having to know the details. Good choices are red bell peppers or tomatoes for red, sweet potato or carrots for orange, spaghetti squash or pineapple for yellow, kale or broccoli for green, blueberries for blue, and eggplant for purple.

3. **Buy (some) organic.** Although opting for organic produce is desirable, it is often not economically feasible or readily available. If you know fruits and vegetables have been exposed to many pesticides, purchase organic ones instead. Each year the Environmental Working Group (EWG) puts out a list of the "Dirty Dozen" (high pesticides) and the "Clean Fifteen" (low pesticides). EWG found that by avoiding the 12 most contaminated fruits and vegetables, you can reduce your pesticide exposure by 90%. Buy organic apples, bell peppers, cherry tomatoes, celery, cucumbers, grapes, hot peppers, nectarines, peaches, potatoes, spinach, and strawberries. In addition to buying certain organic produce, it is also beneficial to buy organic baby food, dairy, eggs, meat, peanut butter, coffee, and wine.

4. **Buy local.** Even organic food could have traveled thousands of miles to get to you. On average, the food we eat travels 1,500 miles before it finds its way on to our dining table, depleting nutrients along the way. Local food is picked when it is ripe and is much fresher when you eat it. The best place to find local food is at your farmers market. Be sure to ask if the produce has been sprayed with pesticides or the soil treated with fertilizer. Of course, the most local you can get is by growing your own food! This way you know for sure what you are eating.

5. **Skip the bad fats.** Avoid foods with trans fats and hydrogenated oils. These ingredients are used to extend the shelf life of food, but can be harmful to your health. Studies have linked these fats and oils with heart disease, bad cholesterol (LDL), and obesity.

6. **Play detective.** Consider the food a dessert if it has sugar in the first three ingredients. Sugar is in most packaged foods. There are over 40 names for sugar. It can be disguised as (high fructose) corn syrup, glucose, fructose, dextrose, brown rice syrup, fruit juice concentrate, and evaporated cane juice. No matter what it is called, it is sugar. As you start to pay attention to the labels, you will notice that your salad dressing, ketchup, and jam are all desserts. Use these products mindfully.

7. **Start the day right.** Eating breakfast has many health benefits including increased energy, improved mood, better concentration, and weight control. An egg scramble with spinach and a side of blueberries is a great way to start the day because you get a good mix of proteins and carbs to sustain your energy. Try to avoid sugary, nutrient-free cereals which may give you a quick energy boost, but will soon have you reaching for unhealthy pick-me-ups like sweet treats and caffeinated beverages. If you rely on a cup (or more) of coffee to jumpstart to your day, try eating well, reducing stress, and getting more sleep, instead. These three things will give you more energy than your cup of joe, with the high lasting all day.

8. **Carry snacks.** Regulating your blood sugar throughout the day is critical for your health and will help keep you from

reaching for junk food. If you have healthy snacks with you, you will be less tempted to buy unhealthy food on the go. I carry a homemade trail mix of almonds, walnuts, sunflower seeds, pumpkin seeds, dried cranberries, and dried blueberries. It is good to have a little bit of protein with every meal and snack for blood sugar regulation. Good proteins include lean meats, eggs, beans, lentils, nuts, and seeds.

9. **Go unconventional.** The diet of the animals we eat is important because that is what we are putting into our bodies. Non-organic meat and dairy products can have traces of hormones and antibiotics from treating the animals as they are raised. Drinking milk and eating meats with genetically engineered growth hormones have been linked to colon, breast, and prostate cancers. Conventional factory animals are fed corn and grain instead of grass so they grow faster. They are often given hormones, protein supplements, and antibiotics so they can be slaughtered at younger ages, thus making them more profitable. If you do eat meat, it is best to buy pasture-raised chickens and grass-fed beef. They have much healthier types of fat (more omega-3s), higher levels of vitamins and antioxidants, and no hormones or antibiotics.

10. **Know your fish.** Chemicals from our food, cleaning products, and medications end up in our waterways. Fish swim in the waterways and we eat the fish. This means we are ingesting these chemicals which is not good for our health. Mercury and PCBs (polychlorinated biphenyls) are two of the most significant contaminants. To avoid mercury, eat smaller fish. To avoid PCBs, eat less fatty fish. Buy sustainably

caught seafood—meaning there was no overfishing or destructive fishing methods. The Monterey Bay Aquarium puts out a Seafood Watch guide that you can download from their website to help you chose ocean-friendly seafood.

11. **Eat for yourself.** There are many differing beliefs out there on the "right" way to eat. People can be very passionate and opinionated about it. All sides have research to show why their way is the healthiest way. Some people choose not to eat meat or dairy. Others choose not to eat grains or legumes. Both groups say they feel healthier than ever on their chosen diet. Do your own research and eat the foods that make *you* feel the best. From there, opt for the best quality.

12. **Follow the 80/20 rule!** Eat healthy 80% of the time. This tip is very important—so important that it has an entire chapter about it, *Living in the 80s.* Pleasure is a part of health and we derive pleasure from the food we eat. Do your best to eat well most of the time. When you are dipping into the 20%, just be mindful and savor every bite.

To compliment the 12 tips for eating, here are the top two tips for drinking:

1. **Fill up on water.** Every system in our body depends on water. Water flushes toxins out of our vital organs and carries nutrients to our cells. Lack of water can lead to dehydration, as well as other health issues. A general rule of thumb is to divide your weight by two and drink that many ounces of water each day. For example, if you weigh 140 pounds, you should drink approximately 70 ounces of water

daily. This amount may vary depending on how active you are, the climate you live in, or your health status. Foods can provide some of your water intake (primarily through fruits and vegetables), but it's always good to have water by your side throughout the day. If you don't like the taste of water, try adding lemon, cucumber, mint, or strawberries to give it a little flavor.

2. **Skip the soda.** Soda has no nutritional value and can lead to obesity, type 2 diabetes, and other chronic conditions. Diet sodas may have fewer calories, but they contain artificial sweeteners such as aspartame. Aspartame is believed to cause side effects like headaches, dizziness, mood changes, and loss of memory. Regular sodas may not have artificial sweeteners, but they have empty calories and often contain natural sugars like high fructose corn syrup, which has its own host of health consequences. Giving up or reducing your soda intake can be a huge boost to your health. I like soda as much as the next person (Diet Coke, if you please), but the more I learn about it, the more I skip it. I strongly encourage you to do the same.

There is a lot of noise and confusion out there about how to eat healthy. Follow the tips above and you can't go wrong.

Are you ready to choose a nutrition plan that stands the test of time? If so, it's time to try fad-free eating. Which of the ideas are you already doing and which ones can you incorporate into your life?

24

Pink Ribbons and Red Hearts

What would you do if you were told that you had an 87% chance of getting cancer?

a. fear it

b. ignore it

c. beat the odds!

Fifteen years ago, doctors told me that I had an 87% chance of getting breast cancer because of my genetic predisposition to the disease. I was given a "riskometer" chart (yes, that is actually the title on the chart) with a thermometer-like visual showing which risk factors applied to me and where they fell on the high to low risk range for getting the disease. I was also shown my family tree with many colored in circles and squares of my cancer-stricken relatives. All I could see in my mind was a bunch of pink ribbons and red hearts for the many relatives who had breast cancer on my mom's side (nine accounted for) and heart disease on my dad's side (eight accounted for).

With the statistics quoted to me, the odds seemed stacked against me. Or were they? I had no idea where these numbers came from and what they really represented. What was the sample size? How long ago was the study done? Did they look at diet and lifestyle to see if these correlated at all to whether or not people got the disease? What would the study results have been if they only included people who had the genetic predisposition *and* lived a healthy lifestyle? Perhaps then the statistics quoted to me by the doctors would have been a little less daunting.

People often make serious health and life decisions based on the statistics they are given, so it's best to do a little digging first to really understand the numbers. When I dug into the 87% statistic quoted to me, I found out that this number came from an older, smaller study. More recent studies have been done with thousands of women that are more reflective of the high-risk population as a whole. One such study showed the lifetime risk to be 65%. A meta study (analysis of several studies) showed the risk to be 57%. Authors of one of the newer studies noted that even these numbers were likely to be overestimates because of the high-risk self-selection process of volunteers to participate in the study. They said the true risk could be as low as 50%.

It gets confusing, right? It took me a lot of time to read the various studies and understand the numbers. It is important because the choice I make believing I have a 50% risk may be very different than the choice I make with an 87% risk. We are a data-driven society. I'm left-brained and I like numbers as much as the next person. You'll see in this book that I often quote statistics to illustrate a point. I've done my best to quote from reputable sources. Still, I've seen all too often where, over time, a statistic becomes an accepted fact with the truth of the source no longer referenced, applicable, or current.

The point of all of this: Don't take numbers at face value.

When doctors gave me my odds, I felt as if that was how they were defining me. They didn't know anything about me other than my genetic makeup and family history. Yet all sorts of assumptions were made about me and, consequently, about the course of action I should take like preventative surgeries and toxic medications. When I first was given this statistic, I operated out of fear, seeing myself as a pink ribbon and red heart waiting to happen. After time, I ignored the statistic. And, finally, I decided it was time to move from fear to empowerment and beat the odds! As I researched, I discovered the science of epigenetics which shows that genes are not our destiny. There are other influencing factors including how we live our life—the foods we eat, how much we exercise, the way we manage our stress, the environment we live in, and so on.

The pink ribbons and red hearts are only a part of who I am. They are counterbalanced (and then some!) by all of the healthy influences in my life—running the trails with my dog, laughing with friends, eating fresh tomatoes from the garden, traveling to new lands, snuggling with my cat, riding my cruiser bike, relaxing in the backyard with my husband, taking family vacations, and being alone. All of these things give me health. This is the whole of me.

Don't trust statistics without digging into them further yourself. If you are given odds of getting or surviving a disease, listen to the Dalai Lama when he tells us, *"Tibetans have a saying: If bad news comes, you listen here (points to the right ear) and let it out here (points to the left ear)."* Don't let the statistic take over your mind and become your reality. Focus on creating health in the areas of your life where you can.

Do you have a colored ribbon in your family tree? If so, what are the healthy influences in your life that counterbalance it?

Is Your Body Healthy?

Indicators for health and illness in the Body quadrant focus on our physical health. Diet, exercise, and lifestyle can affect our health. A "yes" answer represents an indicator for health and a "no" for illness, unless otherwise noted.

- Do you do regular physical activity?
- Do you eat fresh, wholesome, real food?
- Do you follow your own healthy diet that is right *for you*?
- Do you drink a lot of water?
- Do you rest when your body is tired?
- Are you rested in the morning when you wake up?
- Do you sleep soundly through the night?
- Do you have energy throughout the day?
- Do you have flexibility in your body?
- Do you use non-toxic beauty products?
- Do you use prescription medications mindfully?
- Do you proactively make your own decisions for health care?
- Are you in tune with your body to know when it is in pain or stressed?
- Do you have pain or physical discomfort? ("yes" is illness indicator)
- Do you eat a lot of sugar, salt, and fatty (processed) foods in your diet? ("yes" is illness indicator)

Guided by the ideas in this section, look at where you answered "no" in the earlier questions and try to identify how these can become "yes." Do the same for the last two questions if you answered "yes" and try to figure out how they can become "no."

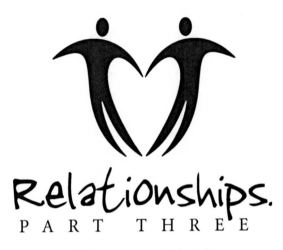

Relationships.

PART THREE

Relationships and Health

Amy dreaded going to work. She liked her job, but her coworker, Joe, made her life miserable. Joe had total disregard for his job. Amy was making the same amount of money as he was for the same work, but he took personal calls and played with his iPad much of the time. It seemed that Joe expected his coworkers to pick up the slack. He was also a bully. Anytime Amy had a personal conversation with a coworker, he would make snide comments. If she laughed, he would copy her with a mocking laugh. In order to avoid giving Joe something to ridicule, Amy began to keep to herself.

Beaten down at work, Amy sought comfort by indulging in the unending sugary treats she found in the break room. She was so drained at the end of the day, that she would typically come home and watch hours of television. She wasn't motivated to do any exercise and she rarely saw her friends anymore. She was stressed, depressed, and had low self-esteem. She was also overweight and had high blood pressure.

The Relationships quadrant represents our personal connections to others and to the larger culture and society. We need to put the same kind of energy into actively managing our relationships that we do into eating right, exercising, reducing stress, and creating a healthy environment. Research shows that people with a strong social network live longer and are healthier than those without supportive people in their lives. Having strong relationships has been shown to decrease depression, increase self-esteem, and promote better stress management.

There are many ways to create stronger relationships, such as identifying your emotional triggers, as discussed in the chapter *Trigger Happy*. When you do not resolve issues from your past, it can undermine your new relationships. Another way to build stronger bonds, as discussed in *Freaky Friday*, is to try to understand the other person's perspective.

Just as having strong relationships can boost your health, having weak or no relationships can harm your health. Living in isolation and surrounding yourself with negative influences have been shown to raise blood pressure, affect sleep quality, and increase production of the stress hormone cortisol. As discussed in *Exiting Stage Left*, it is important to actively manage your social network so that you spend less time with people who deplete you and more time with those who lift you up.

Amy's relationship with Joe definitely had an impact on her health. It drained her energy and lowered her self-esteem, keeping her in a constant state of stress. She felt isolated at work because she couldn't talk to her coworkers without Joe ridiculing her. This isolation carried into her personal life too because she was feeling so low about herself.

After recognizing the influence Joe was having on her health, Amy decided it was time to take back control. She visualized a "shield" around Joe and imagined that all of his negativity stayed within that shield. After practicing this image, Amy took it with her to work. When Joe would make a comment, the remark would bounce off the shield and stay in his orb, not entering hers at all. With this new sense of empowerment, one day when Joe was mocking her, Amy brusquely told him to stop. Perhaps it was the force in her voice or the way she now carried herself, but, to her surprise, it worked. Joe seldom makes comments to her anymore. Amy no longer feels isolated—at work or at play.

Because she no longer has Joe bringing her down, Amy has quickly made amazing strides in other areas of her life. She joined a gym and eats healthier. She has gone down two belt sizes and has lowered her blood pressure. She spends time with her friends and family. Amy feels like a completely different person now that she is spending less energy on Joe and more on herself and those who support her.

Dr. Dean Ornish, who has had great success with the reversal and prevention of heart disease in his 30 years of directing clinical research, believes that love and intimacy are among the most powerful factors in health and illness. He says, "I am not aware of any other factor in medicine—not diet, not smoking, not exercise, not stress, not genetics, not drugs, not surgery—that has greater impact on our quality of life, incidence of illness, and premature death from all causes." That's a pretty powerful statement.

There are many ways to manage and deepen your relationships, a few of which have been highlighted above. You'll also read about resisting the temptation to allow technology to be a third party in your relationships and reconnecting through touch. In addition, you'll learn how helping your community and spending time with your pets is good for your health.

Read on to learn about changes you can make in your Relationships to promote your overall health.

25

Exiting Stage Left

Imagine this…You are upset because you had a conflict with your boss. You have a lunch date scheduled with your friend, Susie, that you want to cancel but she insists on meeting because she wants to hear about it. As soon as she sees you, she gives you a hug. She immediately asks you what is going on. She listens intently while you tell your story. You get so worked up that you start to cry. Susie puts her hand on yours, and tells you to go on. When you are finished relating your story, Susie says she understands why you are so upset. She asks if you want to brainstorm some ideas about how to handle the situation. After coming up with a few ideas, you start to feel better. By the end of the lunch, you feel energized, supported, and empowered.

Now imagine this instead…You are upset because you had a conflict with your boss. You have a lunch date scheduled with your friend, Michelle, that you want to cancel but she insists on meeting because she wants to talk. As soon as she sees you, she signals that she will be off the phone in a minute. When she finishes her other conversation, Michelle immediately begins to fill you in on her life. Half way into the lunch, you try to share about the conflict with your boss. She says she can relate and tells you about some of her past conflicts with her bosses. When she has finished, you try again to talk about your experience. You get so worked up that you start to cry. Michelle doesn't notice because she is attending to a text that just came through on her phone. Although Michelle asks you to continue, you feel shut down so you say that you are finished. Michelle carries the conversation for the remainder of your time together. By the end of the lunch, you feel sad, lonely, and defeated.

Are you spending more of your time with Susie or Michelle? If it's the latter, it's time for some active friend management. Just as the food we eat, the thoughts we have, and the air we breathe can be toxic, so can the "friends" we keep. The quality of our relationships impacts our health. Friends who are loving, caring, and supportive, like Susie, are good for our health. Friends who are manipulative, mean, or self-absorbed, like Michelle, are not good for our health. A strong social network is about the quality, not quantity, of our friends.

The good news is that we have the power to choose our relationships. The easy test of whether a certain friend is good for your health is to ask yourself whether you feel better or worse after spending time with this person. I have many friends who make me feel wonderful when we spend time together. I get the feeling that they genuinely like me and want to be with me. They are engaged in our conversations and take a sincere interest in what is going on in my life. Our conversations are balanced. They make me feel safe so that I am comfortable sharing my vulnerabilities. Around them, I feel smart, funny, pretty, and likable. I am at my best.

On the flipside, I can identify a couple of people in my life that have made me feel worse after being with them. Becky would either ignore me or make a comment about my personality that felt like an insult. When I spent time with her, I could feel my self-esteem go down. With Steve, I felt that the relationship was unbalanced where I was the giver (listener) and he was the receiver (talker). When I was with him, I could feel my breath rate increase and my muscles tense because he made me feel like he had no interest in what was going on in my life. After our time together, I felt frustrated, drained, and unfulfilled. When I am with people like Becky and Steve, I am more reserved and I feel deflated. I no longer spend time with Becky and Steve.

It may not be easy or comfortable to actively manage your friends, but it is necessary for your optimal health. Going forward, be mindful of the people you spend time with and think about how they make you feel. Exiting stage left from your friends takes conscious effort. It may be a little scary at first, but it will feel liberating once you do it. As you start to realize the impact these people had on you (lowering your self-esteem, causing you stress, bringing you down) and how good you feel without them in your life, you won't settle for anything less. Life is too short to be surrounding yourself with people who drain your energy and deplete your health.

Who in your life thinks the world of you and supports your health? Call them this week to set a date to get together or simply to say "thank you." Who are the people in your life that make you feel worse about yourself by putting you down, talking behind your back, being negative, or making it all about them? For these "friends," it's time to exit stage left.

26

Trigger Happy

One of the best things you can do for your relationships is to identify your triggers. A trigger is an unresolved issue from your past that continues to resurface throughout your life. Think of times in your relationships when you overreacted to a situation—where the reaction you had was way bigger than was warranted for the actual event. In this instance, there likely was a trigger involved.

One of my triggers went off a few months ago when I woke up to find my husband gone from the house. The previous evening we had talked about possibly going to a morning gym class. I woke up a few minutes before the class was set to begin. I was in total disbelief that my husband had gone without waking me to see if I wanted to go. I was seething. I flew out of bed and made it to the gym 10 minutes late. When I got to the class, I marched right over to my husband and made it clear that I was going to use his gym equipment. He would have to miss some of the class to get new equipment for himself. At the time (while triggered), this act seemed completely rational. In hindsight, I see that this was completely reactive, and I realize the power of these unresolved issues.

After class, my husband truly had no idea why I was so upset. He said he had tried to wake me but I did not budge. So, he left. For him, it was as simple as that. For me, it was much more complicated. How could he abandon me? Ah...the trigger. Abandonment.

Yes, I have abandonment issues. My parents divorced when I was three years old. Although both of my parents were active in my life growing up, I still felt abandoned because I did not have the traditional family unit that all of my friends had. I don't think about being abandoned in my daily life. After all, these events happened decades ago. Today, I have a great relationship with my parents who have always been a significant part of my life and who love me very much. I am married to a husband who, I know, will never abandon me.

None of this seems to matter when I wake up that Sunday morning to an empty house and, just like that, I am a three-year-old child feeling abandoned again. My reaction to my husband going to the gym without me was really quite ridiculous. It's easy for me to see this now. However, in the moment, my reaction felt entirely valid, and I was truly angry.

What is your trigger? Is it feeling abandoned? Deprived? Vulnerable? People with abandonment triggers don't trust others to support them. They might react by avoiding close relationships, being clingy, or repeatedly accusing others close to them of being unavailable. They may find ways to drive off normally reliable people, thus making abandonment a self-fulfilling prophecy.

People with deprivation triggers can feel like things are never enough and turn off others with constant demands. They may choose relationships with others who aren't capable of giving care or support.

People with vulnerability triggers have an exaggerated fear that some catastrophe is about to strike. They may be overly conscientious to ensure a feeling of safety. I have only mentioned a few of the triggers here, but there are others. If you are interested in learning more about triggers, I recommend reading Tara Bennett-Goleman's *Emotional Alchemy*.

We react when we are not in touch with our emotions. The

emotions have the power and we have vanished. We are no longer present. In the moment, we can feel like we have no control over what we say or do. The trigger leads the way. In my case, my reaction toward my husband had nothing to do with him. However without this awareness (preferably before the reaction, but after is better than nothing), my relationship could certainly have been affected. By not owning up to our triggers, we bring our past baggage to our current relationships. This isn't fair to our new relationships.

What can we do about our triggers? The best thing to do is to try to sit with the emotion as you are feeling it. Take a few breaths and really feel the emotion. Try to identify where in your body you are feeling the emotion. What is coming up for you? Why are you reacting so strongly? If I had given myself a moment before flying out of the house to really think about what I was feeling and why I was feeling it, I may have been able to understand that old issues were being triggered. I didn't do this. Instead, I reacted.

Awareness is a great first step toward not being trigger happy. The more we can be aware of our triggers, the less likely they are to repeat over and over again throughout our lives—and the healthier our relationships can be.

Next time you experience an especially strong reaction to a situation, try to take a moment to ask yourself if you are being triggered. Can you be aware of the emotion instead of letting it take hold of you?

27

Vitamin T

Let's say you're having coffee with a friend for an hour. How many times do you think you touch her? Believe it or not, the answer varies widely depending on which country you come from. Over the course of an hour, U.S. friends touch each other on average only twice an hour, whereas French friends touch 110 times, and Puerto Rican friends touch 180 times![24] Americans are Vitamin T (touch) deprived—and that could be hurting our health.

Are you getting enough Vitamin T in your life? Natural sources of Vitamin T include handshakes, hugs, kisses, cuddles, and rubs obtained from family and friends. "Vitamin T is absorbed through the skin and helps to soothe the body, calm the mind, warm the heart, and nourish the spirit," say Bob Czimbal and Maggie Zadikov in their light-hearted book, *Vitamin T*. Of course, Vitamin T is not a real vitamin, but calling it out as such underscores the importance of touch in our lives, and studies back this up.

Research shows that lack of touch can lead to decreased emotional health, reduced intellectual ability, and a weakened immune system. On the flipside, having touch in your life can have a variety of health benefits, including decreased breathing rate, reduced muscle tension, lowered resting heart rate, decreased anxiety, increased immune function, increased pain relief, acceleration of wound healing, and relaxation.

The Touch Research Institute, established in 1992 by Tiffany Field at the University of Miami School of Medicine, studies touch and its application in science and medicine. The Institute has conducted over 100 studies on the positive effects of massage therapy. Among the significant research findings are enhanced growth in preterm infants, diminished pain for fibromyalgia sufferers, increased pulmonary function in asthma patients, decreased glucose levels in diabetics, and enhanced immune function for HIV and cancer patients. Many of these effects appear to be mediated by decreased stress hormones.

There are many types of healing touch such as acupressure, reflexology, Jin Shin Jyutsu, and massage. The chapter *Four-Legged Therapy* highlights the health benefits of cuddling with our pets. When we come in contact with another being—pet, loved one, or healing practitioner—beta-endorphins, a natural morphine-like substance, are released by the brain into our blood stream which improves our mood, among other health benefits noted above.

Candace Pert, neuroscientist and key figure in the discovery of the endorphin molecule, says, "From my research with endorphins, I know the power of touch to stimulate and regulate our natural chemicals, the ones that are tailored to act at precisely the right times in exactly the appropriate dosages to maximize our feelings of health and well-being." Clearly, there are beneficial physiological and psychological responses that happen in our bodies and minds when we touch. Touching is a great way to experience a natural high.

Even if touchy feely isn't your style, try adding a little more touch into your life. Give more hugs, hold hands with your spouse, console a friend with an arm on her shoulder. Forget the air kisses and go for the full on bear hugs. It's a pretty fun and easy way to get more health into your life.

Where do you fall on the touchy feely scale and how can you get more Vitamin T in your life?

28

Me, You, and "i"

I'd like to introduce you to my faithful pal, "i." He's very good at keeping me connected. I rely on him tremendously and find it hard to believe there was ever life without him. I spend more time with him than anyone else. When I ask my husband, "Where is 'i'"?, he knows I am not losing my grammatical skills or waxing philosophical. It means I'm looking for my 4.9" x 2.3" constant companion. "i" is how I lovingly refer to my iPhone. He's here with me now.

As much as I love "i," I'm feeling a bit on information overload at the moment. At our fingertips 24/7, there are beeps, vibrations, and visual notifications that there is something new awaiting our attention. There are numerous conduits of the information—iPhones, Droids, Blackberrys, iPads, laptops, and PCs. There are many ways to transmit the information—email, texting, and blogging. And, there are several social media platforms to engage with, such as Facebook, Twitter, LinkedIn, YouTube, and Pinterest.

I'm all for technology, but at what point does it start to take over our lives? Do you find yourself on vacation trying to get just the right photo to post on your Facebook page instead of truly savoring the moment? Do you text (or worse—answer your cell phone!) when you are spending time with a friend or spouse? Do you spend hours on email, taking away time from loved ones? It seems like it's no longer enough to simply "love the one you're with."

My friend, Lanny, spends miles on his runs crafting witty Facebook status updates. Tiffany gave up Twitter for Lent. As I'm writing this chapter, Samantha is spending the day with her boyfriend. In the past four hours, she has posted 10 times on Facebook. There were eight check-ins and two photos. I know exactly where Samantha was on her date today—where they ate, where they hiked, what bridge they took to get there, and more.

The technological clutter in our lives can be as damaging to our health as the physical clutter. It takes away from time that could be spent with others and compromises the serenity in our lives. What is your technological drug of choice? Is it posting frequently on Facebook, texting constantly, or perusing YouTube?

I have to be honest with you because we're coming clean with each other and facing our technological addictions together. Throughout the writing of this chapter, I have deleted 54 emails and sent 23. Each time I get a new email, I get a visual notification at the bottom of my screen that lures me away from the task at hand. I wonder how much more productive I could have been if I had turned the notification off and checked my emails when I was done.

I'm not asking you (or myself) to quit cold turkey, but are there one or two changes you can make to help quiet your mind and nurture quality relationships? Here are seven ideas.

1. **Reduce emails.** For personal emails, which distribution lists can you unsubscribe to? Do you really need the daily coupons and marketing announcements from stores or numerous notifications of travel deals? Oftentimes, you have been added to a list without your knowledge. At the bottom of most mass emails, there is an "unsubscribe" link that you can click on. For work emails, request not to be copied on communications you don't need to be. Ask or answer questions in person or over the phone so that you don't end up going back and forth in numerous emails.

2. **Delete, not forward.** Do us all a favor, if you get a chain email, don't forward it to your entire email distribution list. Use discretion on when and to whom you forward it. Make sure it's really funny, poignant, or important. If it's not, take one for humankind and delete it from cyberspace.

3. **Help yourself.** Silence the visual or auditory notification on your cell phone and computer so that you aren't tempted with every email, text, or Facebook update you get.

4. **Be present.** When you are with others, leave your cell phone ringer off and put it in your purse or pocket. Make it a table for two, not three. Resist the temptation to do a quick text or answer the phone while you're having dinner with a good friend (unless you think it's an emergency, of course). Be present with the one you are with; the others can wait.

5. **Play the game.** A good way to accomplish the previous idea is to play the Phone Stack game. When out to lunch or dinner with friends, everyone puts their phones face down at the center of the table upon arrival. Whoever is the first one to give in to the temptation of the various buzzes and rings signaling texts, emails, and calls, pays the bill. If no one reaches for the phones, you split the bill.

6. **Disconnect.** When you are on vacation, try to disconnect. See if you can go without email, Facebook, and/or Twitter— even if it's just for one day. You don't even have to be on vacation, try it on a weekend day.

7. **Ask why.** Ask yourself why you feel the need to be so tied to your _____ (fill in your social network of choice). Is it filling

a void? Is it giving you something you are not otherwise getting in your relationships? Are you bored? Is it a compulsion (e.g. the need to have an empty in-box)? Spending time thinking about why you are doing it could lead to some personal insights.

When your connection with technology is coming from a healthy place and there is balance, that's great. I am a big fan of technology and social media. Facebook has allowed me not only to reconnect with many old friends, but also to keep up with my current friends. I've seen the power of LinkedIn firsthand, with a friend of mine recently getting a job through one of my connections. This chapter is not about technology or social media bashing. It's about finding the balance.

When it gets to the point where technology takes over your mind and/or infringes on time with your loved ones, it's time for an intervention. Last night, I was rubbing my husband's head with one hand as he fell asleep because he was feeling stressed. With the other hand, I was emailing. That's when it hit me that maybe I needed to set some boundary limits with "i."

Do you need to set some boundaries with your technology friends to nurture the health in your Mind and Relationships quadrants?

29

Find Your People

It's nine o'clock on a Tuesday night and I'm at a veterinary hospital to meet a dog that I might adopt. This particular vet works a lot with rescue organizations. The rescue group that I contacted told me that I could meet the dog before she got spayed if I came that evening. It seemed a little late to me, but the dog had just been listed online at Petfinder and I found myself saying "yes." As I waited to meet the dog, I saw multiple rescue groups come in and out with animals that needed help. It was amazing to me that the vet's office was hopping so late at night.

As I sat and watched these rescue people do their work, I thought to myself, "I get it." I get why they are here working so hard. I understand that it doesn't matter that it's late; these lives need to be saved. I'm an animal person. I have always had a soft spot for cats and dogs. When I married my husband, I had one condition: I would always have at least one four-legged companion in my life (up until this night, it had been cats).

As I waited to meet my future pup (yes, it was an instant love connection), I thought that some people might look at these volunteers and not really get it. Why would someone willingly be out so late to help a dog or cat they didn't even know? As I sat there, I had this feeling come over me that these are "my people." I ended up staying there until midnight, offering to photograph the just-rescued shelter animals so they could be posted online for faster adoption.

Who are "your people"—the people who understand your

passion and beliefs without your even having to say a word? These are the people to whom you can relate completely. You can be authentic around them, not having to pretend to be someone else or downplay who you are. Is it your fellow cyclists? A knitting group? Cancer survivors? Church members? A new mom's group? Foodies?

Now that I'm a new dog owner, I'm seeing that I have another group of new "people." There is a whole subculture when you own a dog that I previously had no idea existed. In the two years that I've had Kora, I've connected with dozens of new people. I started a blog about being a new dog mom to a high-energy border collie mix and I have people chiming in from all parts of the world. Our dogs instantly connect us.

It's the same for runners too. I know before I started running, I didn't know about "the runner's wave"—the acknowledgement that we are kindred spirits. I regularly walked the same path that I now run on, but I was never privy to this secret sign between runners until I went out for my first run.

I can imagine it's also true for foodies, like my friend Doug. He loves to talk food. Whereas I might say, "We had a delicious salmon and asparagus dinner last night," Doug gives a 20-minute explanation about how the meal was prepared (down to the ingredient list and steps). I always wonder if Doug knows I'm not actually retaining any of his food reviews. I'm guessing another foodie would be interested in the details and be able to replicate the meal later on.

The point is, spending time with your people—the people who get who you are at some fundamental level—allows you to be authentic. You don't have to feel like you need to hide a part of yourself or downplay something you are passionate about. It's okay if you talk for 30 minutes about the woes of your running feet or tell stories of how your dog is the cutest and smartest dog ever. They get it. Spending time with your people is good for your health.

Who are your people and do you spend enough time with them? If not, how can you make more of an effort to do so?

30

Crazy Runner Girl

Anne Mahlum was just a girl who ran. She would run by a homeless shelter every day in her hometown of Philadelphia and see the men outside on the corner. The homeless men would shout out to her, calling her "crazy runner girl."

One morning, Anne wondered why she was the runner and they were the homeless. She thought, "Why can't we all just be runners?" From this question, she started Back on My Feet (BOMF), encouraging the homeless men to join her in training for a half marathon.

The program grew from there. Starting just a few years ago in July 2007, the organization is now operating in 11 cities and works with many shelter facilities. BOMF is more than about encouraging homeless men to run. It's about promoting self-sufficiency by engaging these individuals in running as a means to build confidence, strength, and self-esteem. In the six years of operation, over 600 members have obtained housing, 900 have secured jobs, and 630 have enrolled in job training programs—all of this from one woman's thought while out on a run.

Anne Mahlum was just a crazy runner girl who decided to make a difference. Now she is an agent for change, using running to connect people. She says, "There are so many differences between all of us, but running reminds us just how similar we are. When we run, there is no separation between race, gender, age, or socioeconomic status." Through her actions, she promotes health for individuals and for her community.

Recently in my neighborhood there was a group home for juvenile kids on probation. My neighbors were not happy about it. They rallied and spoke at a city meeting to try to get the kids out of the home to make it a single family home again. I tried to explain to my neighbors that perhaps instead of chasing the kids out, we could welcome them into the community. I even considered creating a running program for them, similar to BOMF.

I encountered a lot of resistance. I did not act to make my community a better place. I let fear and opposition prevent me from action. The group home has since been moved out of the area. I hope next time the opportunity presents itself, I choose to step up to the plate and make a difference.

We can get so caught up in our own lives that we operate from a self-centered mindset. Oftentimes, our mindset expands to include our family and friends into our circle of care and concern. Ideally, our view expands even further to include compassion for all people. From this wide view, we are able to see the shared commonalities among us. We connect on a human level, regardless of race, sex, religion, and ethnicity.

Helping others has health benefits for you, too. Research shows that people who volunteer have greater longevity, higher functional ability, lower rates of depression, and less incidence of heart disease. Volunteering gives you a sense of purpose and helps you feel connected with others. You may even experience a "helper's high" from the release of endorphins (feel good hormones) in your body. When we make our community healthier, we make ourselves healthier. And, when we make ourselves healthier, we make our community healthier.

Grassroots efforts *can* (and do!) make a difference. Fortunately, there are many people like Anne Mahlum in this world who have shown how the power of one can amplify for the good of many.

How can you make your community (and the world) a healthier and better place—and in the process boost your own health?

31

Four-Legged Therapy

Who in your life provides you with unconditional love, greets you with pure joy, appreciates the time you spend with them, encourages you to exercise and get outside, makes you feel needed and important, and snuggles at will? In my life, it has been Oreo, Spanky, Alfalfa, Hollywood, and Kora—my four-legged faithful companions.

My pets have given me so much love, happiness, joy, laughter, and health over the years. Even if you are not able to have a pet of your own, you can volunteer at a shelter to take care of the abandoned cats or offer to walk your neighbor's dog. When we spend time with pets, we feel better. Is there a prescription drug that can make us feel as good as a puppy licking our face or a kitten cuddling in our arms?

Because of the love and happiness we feel when we are with our furry friends, it is no surprise that the positive physiological and psychological responses happening in our body include lower resting heart rate, improved mood, lower anxiety, and less loneliness. The benefits don't stop there.

Erika Friedmann, a professor of nursing at the University of Maryland, is a pioneer in researching the relationship between furry companionship and cardiovascular health. She found higher survival rates a year after heart surgery for patients with pets in their homes than for those who had none. She also found that elderly people who own pets visit their doctor less.

In another study of almost 6,000 people by the Baker Medical Research Institute in Melbourne, Australia, results show that pet owners had lower blood pressure and cholesterol levels than did non pet owners, a result that could not be explained by such personal differences as cigarette smoking, diet, weight or socioeconomic profile.

These are just a few of the many studies showing the health benefits of spending time with our four-legged friends. It is no surprise based on these findings that pet therapy programs have popped up across the country. Cats and dogs visit nursing homes and hospitals to help patients feel better and heal faster.

Some dogs are even trained to help people with certain health issues, such as diabetes, seizures, autism, and pain. For example, a diabetic alert dog notices the chemical changes that occur in its owner's body as blood sugar drops and notifies the owner by barking or licking. Seizure dogs bark to alert others when their owner is having a seizure and can even retrieve the phone for a 911 call.

Mahatma Gandhi said, *"The greatness of a nation and its moral progress can be judged by the way its animals are treated."* In this country, we run the gamut. At one end, there are animals that are treated like family members, their every need thoughtfully attended to. At the other end, there are blatant acts of cruelty against animals like hoarding, puppy mills, dog fighting, and worse. Last year, I read about 15 small dogs that were intentionally dumped in the middle of a busy road, some hit by cars not able to stop in time. There is no excuse for the inhumane treatment of animals. When we hurt others, including animals, we hurt ourselves.

Animals don't speak our language. They are dependent on us for their needs—food, water, shelter, and love. We have to be their advocates. It is a big responsibility and one that should not be taken lightly.

Do you have a furry friend that lights up your life? If so, go give them a hug and thank them for promoting your health.

32

Do You Know?

Do you know what your spouse believes to be the meaning of life? Do you know how old your parents think they would be if they didn't know how old they were? Do you know your sibling's life motto?

These are a few of the questions that I posed to my family this past Thanksgiving. I created a document with 13 questions and asked my family to fill it out a few days before the holiday. After dinner, we went through each of the questions trying to figure out who said what. It was fun, heartwarming, and informative. Here are the questions.

1. If you were stranded on an island, what three foods and one drink (other than water) would you want an unlimited supply of?

2. If you were featured on the cover of a magazine, which one would you want it to be?

3. What are the place(s) you still want to travel to that you have not (assuming perfect health and you had the money)?

4. What is a food or drink that you miss that you have given up for health reasons?

5. What is your favorite quote?

6. What is your life's motto?

7. What are you most proud of in your life?

8. What were the defining moments in your life (i.e. changed the course of your life)?

9. What is the meaning of life?

10. Name a funny word.

11. If the ATM gives you $1,000 instead of $100, what would you do?

12. If you could re-name yourself, what would it be?

13. How old would you be if you didn't know how old you were?

How often do you talk about these kinds of questions with your friends and family? Too often we are caught up in reporting what is going on for us (or others) and that drives our conversations. There is nothing wrong with this, but sometimes it is a good change of pace to talk about broader and deeper life topics. You may learn a few things that you didn't know about your loved ones.

A few years ago, *Table Topics* cards came out which are great conversation starters for intimate dinners for two or large parties. *Talk to Me* by Bonnie Sose and *The Book of Questions* by Gregory Stock have hundreds of questions covering a wide range of topics.

Taking it one step further, you can buy a family member *The Story of a Lifetime* by Pamela and Stephen Pavuk. It is a beautifully bound book with hundreds of questions covering all areas of life. There is room in the book to write the answers, so it is a great keepsake once completed. My sister and I gave the book to my dad several years ago. He worked on it for two years to complete it. This is something I will cherish forever. If your loved ones do not want to do it on their own, you can interview them in short sessions to capture the information.

I have also recorded several of my family members answering some of the questions. When our loved ones are no longer physically with us, one of the things we miss is the sound of their voice. To have these recordings means a lot to me because I know that I will be able to hear their voices forever. You can buy (or borrow) a digital recorder and then save it on your computer. Many smart phones have recording capability as well. I know "i" does.

Getting to know my friends and family on a deeper level has helped me to create special bonds. I loved learning that my 71-year-old mom feels like she is 60, and that my husband thinks the meaning of life is to "Leave the world a better, happier place than when you entered it."

Do you know what your friends would re-name themselves if given the chance? If not, it may be fun to find out.

33

"I Think I'm in Love"

My good friend, Beth, recently said to me, "I think I'm in love." I have to admit—I felt a twinge of jealousy. I knew how she was feeling in that moment. Do you remember that "in love" feeling when you feel like you are on cloud nine? All is right with the world and you feel positively aglow. You want to spend every moment with your new seemingly soul mate. The relationship is so new that you have no responsibilities within it. There are no bills to pay together, no kids demanding attention, no house that needs upkeep, and no outside interested parties involved. The relationship is just between you and your newfound partner.

I've been with my husband, Dave, for 26 years, married for 17. I love my husband and our life together. I truly feel that he loves me unconditionally, and I wouldn't trade it for anything. However, like most long-term partnerships, our relationship now comes with responsibilities and a never ending to-do list. Richard Carlson, in his *Don't Sweat the Small Stuff… and It's all Small Stuff*, said, "Remind yourself that when you die, your 'in-basket' won't be empty." I read this book over a decade ago yet these words still stay with me. We can't (always) let the overflowing inbox be an excuse not to do something fun with our loved one.

How do we keep the spark alive and have that "in love" feeling again? Here are five suggestions.

1. **Make time.** Yes, this is difficult with all of the demands on our time—work, children, friends, and family. However,

our relationships are worth leaving the to-do list undone periodically. If it helps to schedule the time like you do other appointments, do it.

2. **Touch more.** The chapter *Vitamin T* discussed how disconnected physically to each other we are as a nation. You can always spot a newly in love couple because they seem to be in constant physical contact with one another. As our relationships progress, we seem to lose this connection. Make an effort to hold hands, give hugs, and put your arms around your significant other.

3. **Greet with a wag.** Recently my friend, Bev, was remembering her beloved dog that died a year ago. She was talking about all that she learned from him. She said she loved the way he always greeted her when she came home. Dogs reliably greet us with such pure glee and affection when we walk through the door. Bev said that she tries to do this with her husband every day. I love this idea. I'm usually working on the computer when Dave gets home. I have one last bit of work that I want to get done until I am ready to engage, which typically ends up taking much longer than I had anticipated. I definitely do not greet him like our dog, Kora, greets him. Thanks, Bev, for the inspiring idea that will bring a smile to many surprised partners coming home. I know Dave appreciates the new daily homecoming ritual.

4. **Get to know.** In the previous chapter, *Do You Know?,* you read about connecting on a deeper level. Ask some of the questions featured and you may discover something new about your loved one that you didn't know.

5. **Have fun.** Think about what you enjoyed doing together when you first met. My husband and I loved to play pinball together with him operating the left flipper and me at the right. What was it for you? Was it a hike and a picnic, trying out a new recipe cooking together, or exploring a nearby town? You don't even have to go anywhere. You can enjoy your own backyard or sit by the fire in your house, as long as you are doing nothing but being together. Remember, this is not a time for updating each other about the house, children, or job. Nor is it a time to discuss issues that need to be worked out. This is a time for being present with each other, having fun, remembering why you fell in love in the first place, and truly connecting with each other.

Whatever phase you are in with a relationship, appreciate it for where it is. Every stage has its highlights and lowlights. If you are not currently in a relationship, enjoy your time alone doing things for yourself. If you are in a new relationship with that "in love" feeling, savor and appreciate every minute. If you are in a long-term relationship, be grateful for the comfort of enduring and deep love.

What steps can you take to get that "in love" feeling again in your relationship?

34

There is No There

I need to take current event news in small doses. Years ago, I stopped getting the newspaper. I no longer watch the news at night. There are plenty of good things happening in the world, but the news tends to focus on the bad—that's what sells. I find that my heart is too heavy when I open myself up to unlimited reports of tragedy. I still keep in touch—hearing the highlights from my husband, my friends, the radio, and the Internet. I know enough of what I need to know.

When the earthquake and resulting tsunami first hit Japan in 2011, my husband and I watched it on the news. While he sat glued to the television for the next few hours as the devastation unfolded, I stopped watching. I knew that eventually I would see the images and read the stories. It had to be on my own time.

What happened in Japan was overwhelming. First, the country got hit with a 9.0 earthquake, which was the world's fourth biggest earthquake since 1900. As if this weren't enough, a tsunami resulted from the shaken earth—rippling throughout the world. On top of all this, Japan faced radioactive steam leakage from one of its nuclear power plants. Furthermore, with all of this happening in the winter, temperatures hit below freezing. The death toll was estimated at over 15,000.

Whether you are like me and take the news in small doses or someone who watches it all at once, one thing is clear. There is no there. It's all here. What happens 5,000 miles away, like what happened in Japan, may seem like something that is happening "there." However, it is impacting every "here" in the world. We truly are all interconnected in so many ways. When the tsunami happened, global stock markets dropped. Coastal lands thousands of miles away were impacted when the tsunami waves hit the shores of northwestern Canada, the western U.S., Mexico, and more. One person even died in the U.S. from the tsunami that originated thousands of miles away.

The impact is not just limited to external things like drops in the financial market and waves hitting our coastal shores. It also hits us internally. Seeing abandoned animals, shell-shocked people, and annihilated property affects us. We feel it in our hearts.

What happens to people thousands of miles away is happening to each and every one of us all over the world. Thich Nhat Hanh, one of the best known and most respected Zen masters in the world today, said, in response to the Japan devastation, *"The pain of one part of humankind is the pain of the whole of humankind. And the human species and the planet Earth are one body. What happens to one part of the body happens to the whole body. An event such as this reminds us of the impermanent nature of our lives. It helps us remember that what's most important is to love each other, to be there for each other, and to treasure each moment we have that we are alive. This is the best that we can do for those who have died: we can live in such a way that they continue, beautifully, in us."*

I couldn't agree more. What I realize is that no matter how sad the news has made me over the years, feeling it so deeply has guided me to live my best life. I know that life is short and can be altered in an instant, without warning. We've seen this in the tsunami footage from Japan. We saw it during 9/11 in 2001. We saw it again in Hurricane Katrina's devastation on New Orleans in 2005 and the Haiti earthquake in 2010.

I take Thich Nhat Hanh's words to heart. I choose to honor

the people in Japan, Haiti, New Orleans, and New York by living my best life and creating the life that I want. For me, this means seeking out meaning and being happy, living healthy, surrounding myself with people who love me, and nurturing the world around me. It means living mindfully, appreciating life, and sharing this journey with others.

How will you live your best life to honor the interconnectedness of humankind?

35

Freaky Friday

Do you remember the movie, *Freaky Friday*? It was originally made in 1976 with Barbara Harris and Jodie Foster and redone in 2003 with Jamie Lee Curtis and Lindsay Lohan. The premise of the movie is that a mom and daughter are trapped in each other's bodies and have to switch lives for a day. Previous to the switching, they have little in common and don't get along. After getting a new perspective on the situation by living the other's life for a day, they gain insights into each other. This results in an increase in understanding and respect for one another.

This idea of trying to understand another person's perspective can be very beneficial in relationships. We can't actually switch lives for a day, but we can try to put ourselves in each other's shoes. There is a great way to do this called the 3-2-1 process, as highlighted by Ken Wilber, and his colleagues, in *Integral Life Practice*.

3 – Face It. Think about someone that makes you irritated, angry, or hurt. Write in a journal (or talk to an empty chair) and describe the person in the 3rd person ("he" or "she"). Explain what it is about this person that bothers you. Be honest and describe it in as much detail as possible. Below is an example.

I don't like visiting my sister-in-law because we have nothing in common. I feel like she makes no effort to get to know me. When I am around her, she doesn't ask about what is happening in my life. I often feel invisible. Family is very important to me and it's hard to see why she wouldn't make more of an effort, especially for my husband's sake. She seems to hold grudges.

2 – Talk to It. Here you enter into a simulated dialogue, using the 2ⁿᵈ person pronoun ("you") talking directly to the person. Try to imagine what they would realistically say back to you. Be open.

> *Me: Why don't you try to get to know me?*
> *Her: I'm busy and I don't feel like we have a lot in common.*
> *Me: But we are family, doesn't that count for anything?*
> *Her: Yes, but so many years have passed now and this is just the way it is.*
> *Me: Do you ever think about reaching out and trying again?*
> *Her: Yes, but I don't know how open you are to it and I don't want to be disappointed again.*

1 – Be It. Now it's time to take their perspective and write or speak in the 1ˢᵗ person, using "I." Be the person you have been talking to. See the world, including his or her relationship with you, entirely from the other person's perspective. Make a statement of identification that begins with "I am _____" or "_____" is me.

I am busy and happy with my life. I feel like there is too much water under the bridge. I don't want to be disappointed. Dave is what connects us and I have a good relationship with him. That is enough.

The second part of this step is to imagine that you said this statement, not the other person. This may feel very uncomfortable at first, but go with it and see what comes up for you. How does it feel when you try to apply it to yourself? Is there any part of it that resonates with you? Oftentimes, the things that most bother us about others are actually our own qualities that we are not able to see in ourselves.

This last statement came from my pretending to be my sister-in-law, but now I need to ask if there is any truth in it for me. The answer is yes. I could apply all of that statement to how *I* feel. Once you are able to identify some truth in the statement, see if you can be open to the back-story of your life as to how you got there. For example, as I think about it, my sister-in-law and I both have strong personalities. My husband and I met when we were young—I was 18 years old. She and I didn't connect with each other from the start. I think we never let go of who each of us were 26 years ago. Living several hundred miles away from each other has prevented us from noticing how the other has grown and matured over time. We would likely have a very different relationship if Dave and I met today.

Doing the 3-2-1 exercise can have important positive outcomes. You might no longer feel irritated with the other person and could even feel compassion for them. In addition to impacting your relationships with others, it can also help you gain insights about yourself and make you feel more peaceful, free, and energized.

I did this as a real exercise as I was writing this chapter in the interest of authentic writing. At first when I did the 3-2-1 process, I had the urge to call my sister-in-law and find out her point of view because I wasn't sure if I was capturing how she felt. The more I sat with it, the more I completely felt at peace about it. I think I really was able to see her perspective.

The benefit of the exercise comes whether or not you use it to have a conversation with the other person. It doesn't necessarily lead to action, but it can open doors for communication since you now come from a less reactive and more compassionate place.

Even if you never have the conversation, you still benefit from the exercise by freeing yourself up. I don't know if my relationship with my sister-in-law will ever be where I'd like it to be ideally, but I don't feel the hurt and disappointment that I once did. I hope you will try this exercise. It can be quite powerful.

Is there someone in your life who is a source of sadness, hurt, or anger? If so, try to look at yourself and your relationship from their perspective. Doing so may give you the Hollywood ending you always wanted.

36

Dying Healthy

What is your relationship with disease? For example, if you were told that you had cancer, you would probably tend to think that you were not healthy. However, having cancer and being healthy are not mutually exclusive.

Getting diagnosed with cancer or another disease is difficult, to say the least, but we have a choice. We can be healthy with cancer or unhealthy. It is our whole self—Mind, Body, Relationships, and Environment—that influences our health. If you are putting good food in your body, getting movement when you can, engaging with others, staying positive, you can *have cancer* and *be healthy* at the same time. You are working with your body rather than against it by taking control where you can and nourishing it in the ways it needs to heal itself. If you let the physical disease of cancer bring sourness into your mind, body, relationships, and environment, you are letting the disease take control of your life.

The language we use and the connotations we have to the words certainly impact our relationship with disease. Cancer and dying are not friendly words. When we talk about treating cancer, we often use words like "fight" the disease, "win the war," "destroy" the cancer cells. We see disease as the enemy. But, the reality is that the disease is a part of us. Therefore, seeing it as the enemy is seeing a part of ourselves as the enemy.

A more holistic approach to disease is to work *with* it instead of *against* it. In *Health with a Chinese Twist,* author Dean Black talks about how the Chinese walk a more peaceful path with health. They understand that fighting disease and creating health are two entirely different activities. While opposing comes from fear, creating comes from hope and empowerment.

While cancer seems like more of a scary, in-your-face word, dying is more of a sad, hush-hush word. We see death as somehow separate from life. In our culture, we often avoid those who are dying because it makes us feel uncomfortable or face our own mortality. The dying are in nursing homes or special areas of the hospital. Instead of *fighting* death, we can benefit from *creating* life in every breath that we have.

You can begin to make this shift by talking more openly about the subject, embracing those who are in the final stages of life, and accepting death as a natural part of life. Until we accept all of life, we cannot truly live. Changing our relationship with death can help us live *and* die healthy.

By definition, I am a previvor. A previvor is "a survivor of a predisposition to cancer." Essentially, previvors are people who have not had cancer, but who have a genetic risk of getting the disease. This term was coined in the year 2000 after a community member of a cancer support organization said she "needed a label." In 2007, *Time* magazine declared the term number three on their list of top 10 buzzwords of the year. In 2010, Congress passed a resolution declaring the last Wednesday of each September to be National Previvor Day.

Personally, I have a visceral reaction to this word. I will never call or consider myself a previvor because it makes me feel unempowered—as if cancer is my destiny. Having the predisposition to cancer is a part of who I am. It's not something I need to "survive" from. This is just another example of how our use of language shapes our relationship with disease and health.

As mentioned earlier in the book, the "nocebo" effect is when a negative health condition is caused by the expectation of that health condition. For example, women who were afraid of dying from a heart attack were more likely to do so than women who did not express this fear. As Maharishi Mahesh Yogi said, "*Whatever we put our attention on will grow stronger in our life.*" For me, identifying myself as a previvor puts too much emphasis and focus on the threat of getting the disease. I'd rather put my attention on being positive, happy, and healthy, than on worrying about what might be.

I have the benefit of knowledge about my risk that my sister did not have, and I don't take this lightly. Information is power. I do the preventative screenings that I need to do and I have made changes in my life to give myself the best chance for health. I leave it at that. I don't give it any more attention than it deserves. Where and how intently are you focusing your attention?

The World Health Organization has the following definition of health: "Health is a state of complete physical, mental and social well-being and not merely the absence of disease or infirmity." This is a good definition of health because it goes beyond simply being free of disease.

Don't let your illness (or threat of illness) define you and take over total control of your life. Try these four steps to help change your relationship with disease and dying.

1. **Take a four quadrant perspective.** As discussed in *The Mental in Illness* in Part One, the Mind quadrant, don't let a diagnosis of ill health in one quadrant affect your entire being. By nourishing your health in the areas where you can, you help yourself stay strong and heal quicker. If you have a physical illness (Body), you can do the following to promote health in other quadrants:
   - Lower your stress and stay positive (Mind)
   - Seek out support from your friends and family (Relationships)

- Create a peaceful, safe environment and spend time in nature (Environment)

2. **Watch what you say.** As highlighted above, our use of language does impact our relationship with health and disease. Think about the words you use to talk about your disease. Are you in battle with it? If so, think about creating health instead of fighting disease.

3. **Pick your own label (or not).** Don't let others assign you a label that doesn't feel good to you. Just because others find comfort in calling themselves previvors, cancer survivors, or diabetics, does not mean you have to if it doesn't fit for you. Some people who have had cancer prefer not to use the term survivor because of the implied battle with the disease or because it makes them feel like a victim. Some alternatives they choose are "cancer thrivers," "cancer graduates," or "NED" (no evidence of disease). Some people who have diabetes do not like to be called diabetic because they feel like it defines who they are. They prefer to say they are a "person with diabetes." The point is, be mindful about the labels that others choose for you or you give to yourself. Either go without a label or choose one that feels empowering to you.

4. **Befriend death and disease.** Illness and death are a part of life. By accepting them, we work with, instead of against, them. Openly talk about these topics with your children, spouse, and parents. Broaching the subject takes away its power and mystique. It helps those who are going through the process feel less alienated and more connected.

What steps will you take to change your relationship with disease and dying?

Are Your Relationships Healthy?

Indicators for health and illness in the Relationships quadrant focus on our social health. Love, support, and intimacy with others can affect our health. A "yes" answer represents an indicator for health and a "no" for illness, unless otherwise noted.

- Do you have the support that you need from your friends and family?
- Do you surround yourself with people who make you feel good about yourself?
- Do you spend time with "your people"?
- Do you have love in your life?
- Do you participate in a support group?
- Do you have physical intimacy (some form of touch) in your life?
- Do you volunteer to help others?
- Do you have a wide circle of compassion?
- Do you feel valued, appreciated, and accepted?
- Do you feel engaged with others?
- Do you spend time with pets or children?
- Are you a member of a religious or social organization?
- Do you feel listened to?
- Do you communicate with others on a deep level?
- Do you have someone in whom you can confide?
- Do you feel alone and in isolation? ("yes" is illness indicator)
- Do you spend time with people who deplete you? ("yes" is illness indicator)
- Do you have unresolved triggers from your past? ("yes" is illness indicator)

- Do you spend more time with technology than with human beings? ("yes" is illness indicator)
- Do you let disease take over your life? ("yes" is illness indicator)
- If you are ill, do you feel ashamed (by society) of having the disease? ("yes" is illness indicator)

Guided by the ideas in this section, look at where you answered "no" in the earlier questions and try to identify how these can become "yes." Do the same for the last six questions if you answered "yes" and try to figure out how they can become "no."

Environment.

PART FOUR

Environment and Health

*S*ean loved having his own business selling insurance. He had been in the same office space for 17 years. It was conveniently located a mile from his home. His clients had been visiting him there for years. The building was a bit dated, but the rent was reasonable. Every year when it rained, water would seep into the office. The building had a flat roof, which certainly didn't help the situation. Sean was used to putting out a bucket to collect the water that dripped from the ceiling. Clients would often comment on a musty smell in the office, but Sean never noticed it.

One year, a storm hit with heavy rain. Water poured through the ceiling and filled buckets daily. When the rain subsided, the landlord called in a restoration company to assess and repair the damage. They brought in dehumidifier fans, ripped out the carpeting, and cut out the dry wall. Sean still went to the office and worked around the mayhem. He started to get headaches and have trouble breathing. In the repair process, tests revealed 10 different kinds of mold. Sean *later learned that mold had been detected two years prior when an architect had been brought in to assess plans to revamp the whole center. For at least two years, likely more, Sean had been working in a toxic environment. Once he thought about it, he realized he had been getting sick more frequently over the past few years.*

The Environment quadrant represents the world we live in—natural and constructed, personal and collective. Of the four quadrants, the environment may be the one that we think least relates to our own health. We may see the environment as somehow separate and outside us. But the truth is that we are intimately connected to our environment. We spray food with pesticides and drive cars that produce pollution, which is bad for the environment's health. We then eat these toxic foods and breathe the polluted air, which is bad for our health. To keep ourselves truly healthy, we need to keep the environment healthy.

Scientists have found more than 100 potentially dangerous industrial chemicals and pollutants in the body of the average American.[25] We encounter them everywhere—indoors and outdoors, at work and at home. They are in the food we eat, the clothes we wear, the furniture we sit on, the carpets we walk on, and more. We ingest the toxins in several ways—through our skin, nose, mouth, and ears. Polluted air and water, excessive noise, radiation, hazardous wastes, chemical-laden cleaning products, and pesticides affect us. The result is an accumulation of chemicals that are foreign to our bodies. We can control our exposure to some of these toxins; others we cannot.

According to the World Health Organization, 25% of health problems are caused by environmental factors. Toxins in the environment have been linked to numerous diseases and health conditions, including asthma, allergies, premature birth, learning disabilities, early puberty, diabetes, reduced fertility, and even many cancers.

You *can* do something about this! In the chapters that follow, you'll get ideas and information on detoxifying your environment. *Shoeless Sanctuary* provides ideas for actions you can take in your home environment, such as cleaning with green products, using air purifiers, drinking filtered water, and gardening organically. *Shrinking Your Wasteline* offers ideas for making changes that will have a collective, longer-term impact on your health, such as reducing the use of plastic bottles, carrying reusable shopping bags, and using recycled paper at work. These changes will reduce wastewater and greenhouse gases, which benefits you in the long run. Understanding that our health is connected to the health of the environment helps us to see the direct connection of our actions, whether the benefit is immediate or deferred.

Sean had been getting sick more frequently in the past couple of years, but he had no idea his office environment was harming his health. The mold had been slowly compromising his immune system. When the situation became acute with the exposed floors and walls, his symptoms escalated to headaches and difficulty breathing. Even though the landlord was taking steps to clean up the environment, Sean was upset that he had not been told two years before about the mold detection. He decided to move his office elsewhere, finding a place just as close to home that actually costs less and looks better. He insisted that a mold inspection be done on his new office space before he moved in. Now that Sean understands the impact the environment has on his health, he has taken additional steps like using green cleaning products and buying portable air purifiers for home and work. Being out of the toxic environment has allowed his immune system to be strong once again.

There are many ways to create a healthy environment, a few of which have been highlighted above. You'll also read about decluttering your personal space, reducing holiday waste, eating sustainably, and appreciating nature in all its splendor.

Read on to learn about changes you can make in your Environment to promote your overall health.

37

Green Exercise for the Sole and Soul

Hiking on a warm, sunny day along a trickling stream. Biking on a foggy morning listening to the sound of the wind rustling through the trees. Running through the open trails encountering wild turkeys. This is "green exercise," and it's good for your sole and soul.

Green exercise is any physical activity done in the presence of nature, such as walking, biking, hiking, running, kayaking, and gardening. Exercising in nature improves not only your physical health but also your mental health and overall sense of well-being. A recent multi-study analysis that reviewed 10 studies involving over 1,200 participants shows that even five minutes of exercise outdoors can be beneficial. Participants experienced increased self-esteem, improved mood, and decreased anxiety. It is interesting to note that the presence of water generated greater effects.[26]

When you are exercising outdoors, be sure to unplug. Try to go without listening to your music or talking on the phone. You may notice that when you take off your headset, you instantly feel more connected to the environment. On a warm spring day you might hear the birds chirping, sounding as joyful as you feel with the long-awaited day of sunshine. Relish feeling the warmth of the sun on your body. Smell the fresh blossoms of the awakening spring. Feel a connection to others you encounter along the way through your shared joy of welcoming the new season.

Next time you are debating between exercising inside at the gym and outside in nature, choose the latter. Notice the sights, sounds, and smells around you. Do you hear the laughter of kids playing in the distance? Do you see the beautiful cloud formation in the sky? How does the earth feel beneath your feet? How does the rain, snow, sun, or wind feel on your face? If you bring your faithful four-legged companion along, be present and let him lead the way. We can all take a lesson from dogs on how to truly enjoy a walk outdoors: be excited to go, spontaneously choose your desired path, stop and smell the flowers when the urge strikes, happily greet those you encounter, and look forward to your next outing. Repeat daily.

Green exercise is clearly a four quadrant activity—one that nourishes the body and mind, and connects us to others and the environment. There is beauty in the simplicity of nature as a source of health. It is free, always accessible, and, quite literally, in our own backyard.

How will you nourish your sole and soul with green exercise this week?

38

Shoeless Sanctuary

If you come to our house, you will see that we have a "no-shoe" policy. Though my family thinks it's a bit of a pain to leave their shoes at the door when they come to visit, we do it for a reason—to keep the toxins out and the health in. We don't have control over many of the toxins outside of our home, but we do have control over much of what happens inside our home. Here are eight ideas that can have an immediate impact on making your home a healthy sanctuary for you and your family.

1. **Leave shoes at the door.** This cuts down on dirt and pollutants tracked into your house. Think about all of the places your shoes travel in a day. When you wear them inside your house, you bring all of that into your home—including lawn pesticides, coal tar from asphalt surfaces, lead, and even E. coli. These substances have been linked to cancer as well as neurological and reproductive disorders. Keep the toxins out by taking off your shoes when you get home. If walking barefoot is painful for you, buy comfortable shoes that you wear only inside your house.

2. **Clean green.** Many conventional cleaning products leave indoor air pollution because of the petrochemical VOCs (volatile organic compounds) and synthetic fragrances. These toxins build up in your house each time you use these products. As they evaporate, they can make their way into your body and can be dangerous to your health. See *Vinegar*

and Soda, Please later in this section for more about the negative health impact of these toxins and some ideas on cleaning green.

3. **Limit the leaching.** Don't heat food in plastic containers if they contain BPA (bisphenol A) because it has been found that the BPA can leach into your foods. Ingesting BPA has been linked to cancer, brain damage, fertility problems, and diabetes. It's best to reheat your food in glass, ceramic, or porcelain and to buy BPA-free when buying plastic containers. BPA can also be found in plastic water bottles, metal cans, and baby bottles. When buying canned products, look for companies like Amy's and Eden Foods that use BPA-free cans. Use stainless steel or glass water bottles, opt for fresh food instead of canned, and look for BPA-free bottles for your baby. Also, avoid using plastic wrap for covering your food, especially when heating in the microwave oven. Plastic wrap contains another hormone disrupting chemical known as phthalates which have been linked to asthma and hormonal problems. Instead, buy a BPA-free microwave food cover which has the benefit of being reusable.

4. **Remodel with care.** When it's time to repaint inside your house, consider using latex over oil-based paint because it releases fewer toxins and contains fewer petrochemicals. Choose one of the many brands with low or no VOCs to paint your domain. When it's time to redo the flooring, opt for low VOC finishes. In the kitchen, choose cabinets without formaldehyde. Don't line the cabinets with vinyl shelf paper that can emit harmful phthalates. Instead, try enamel paint for easy cleaning. As you are restocking the

shelves, be sure to replace your non-stick pots and pans (chemicals can leach into the food as you cook) with cast iron and stainless steel ones.

5. **Set bugs free.** Rather than pulling out the Raid for pest control, try capturing bugs and putting them outside to go along their merry way. If you are afraid of bugs like I am, try this method: cover the bug with a small container, slide a thin magazine under the dish, and then run out of the house screaming, freeing the bug when you get outside. You'll feel good for saving a life. If the problem is larger than a bug here and there and you must find a more permanent removal solution, buy food grade Diatomaceous Earth (DE). DE is the fossilized remains of microscopic shells. When these remains come into contact with insects that have an exoskeleton, such as ants, fleas, bed bugs, and roaches, it pierces their shells so the pests die by dehydration. For humans, DE is soft to the touch and is non-toxic. Be careful not to put it where beneficial bugs like ladybugs live.

6. **Get an air cleaner.** I love my HEPA (High Efficiency Particulate Air) cleaner. It captures 99.97% of airborne particles as small as 0.3 microns from air passing through the filter—this means 1.1 billion particles in an area smaller than one square inch. Translation: with the HEPA air filter, you breathe clean air. I can absolutely tell the difference in my house when the air cleaner is running. When I start sneezing, I check my filter, and sure enough it needs to be changed.

7. **Garden organically.** Feed your gardens naturally with compost of lawn, spent plants, and even food scraps (not

meat, oil, or dairy). Find natural ways of removing pests, such as buying and releasing ladybugs or praying mantises to get rid of aphids. Pull weeds rather than spraying them with harsh chemicals (or embrace them for their natural beauty, as discussed later in *Don't Judge a Weed*).

8. **Be quiet.** Every day, we are bombarded by sounds—leaf blowers, lawn mowers, car alarms, barking dogs, traffic, airplanes, and so much more. Noise can impact our health by affecting our sleep, mood, and stress levels. Noise raises our blood pressure and heart rate, causes hormonal changes, and can cause headaches and anxiety. Noise has been linked to tinnitus (a chronic ringing in the ears), irritability, and depression. Make an effort to take a break from the noise you can control. Turn the television and radio off and enjoy the silence. For the noise you can't control, wear earplugs. I'm a big fan of earplugs. In fact, I'm wearing them now to concentrate on writing this chapter. You can wear earplugs on planes, trains, or whenever you need a break from the noise at home or work.

We don't have control over many of the toxins we encounter outside of our home, but we do have a fair amount of control of what happens inside of our homes. What steps can you take to make your home more of a health haven and less of a toxic zone?

39

Free Space, Free Mind

Is your garage so full that you can't park your car in it? Are there piles of papers in your office that prevent you from finding what you need? Do you have magazines from five years ago? Do you keep every gift, even if you don't like it? Is your closet filled with clothes that haven't been worn in years? If you answered "yes" to any of these questions, then perhaps it's time for some spring cleaning, even if it's not springtime. Creating space in your physical environment can improve your mental health. A cluttered environment makes for a cluttered mind.

Think about where you feel most relaxed. Often, it is in an environment that is clean, tidy, and open. Why not create this type of environment where you spend so much of your time—at home. When you have free space, you make way for a free mind.

Those who know me would say that I keep a pretty clean house. I have very little clutter. Every time I bring new belongings into my house, I discard an equal amount of old things I no longer need. For me, the act of getting rid of clutter is very therapeutic. I still laugh at my aunt's comment when she first visited my house, asking, "Where's all of your *stuff*?"

Here are a few ideas for creating some free space in various parts of your home.

Bedroom. Probably the most cluttered place in your bedroom is your closet. Do you wear all of the clothes in your closet? One idea for managing your closet is to place all of your hangers the same way on a certain date. From that date forward, every time you take an item out, return it with the hanger facing the other way. At the end of the year, donate the items that are still facing the original way since it means you haven't worn the item for the entire year.

If you are keeping clothes that are too small in hopes that you will fit into them again, box them up and store them in the garage. If it is motivating for you to see these items, keep one or two in your closet and box up the rest. After a few years, if the clothes are still boxed, it's time to love yourself where you are at and donate the clothes.

Kitchen. Be honest. Do you really need the novelty, once-a-year gadgets that are crowding out your kitchen drawers and cupboards? How often do you use the ice cream maker, pizza stone, bread maker, pasta maker, and heart-shaped cookie cutter? Even for the items you do use, how many cookie sheets, spatulas, and serving dishes do you really need? Keep the ones you use the most, donate the rest. While you are decluttering your kitchen, check out the expiration dates on the food items in your refrigerator and pantry. Toss those past their prime.

Bathroom. How many different kinds of hair products are now piling up on your vanity? How about makeup? Go through the stash and get rid of the beauty products that you know you aren't going to use, even if they are practically new. Many of the items may have reached their expiration, so it might be time to toss them. Beauty products often don't have expiration dates on them, but here are some general guidelines on how long these items last:

- Mascara: 3 to 6 months
- Eye liner: 3 months (liquid) or 2 years (pencil)
- Lipstick: 2 years
- Eye shadow: 6 months (cream) to 2 years (powder)
- Foundation and concealer: 6 to 12 months
- Powder: 6 months to 2 years
- Cleanser and moisturizer: 1 year
- Sunscreen: 1 year

Keep in mind that natural beauty and skincare products spoil faster because they use fewer harmful preservatives. The best way to know if the product is expired is to watch for changes in smell, color, and consistency.

Office. Are your desk and drawers overflowing with papers? If so, take some time to sort through the pile and put some organization to them. Recycle what you don't need, file what you can, and keep out those that require action. On an ongoing basis, try to keep up with where the papers belong before letting them stack up on the desk. To limit paper management altogether, think twice about printing documents that can be stored online. Be sure to have an organized "filing" system online for easy retrieval. Also, consider signing up for paperless statements for your bills.

Garage. If you can't fit your car in the garage, it's time for some cleaning. What is in all of those boxes stored in the garage? Do they go years without being opened and do you even remember what is in them? Go through the boxes and mark today's date (or the date you store a box, moving forward). If you don't open the box for a couple of years, consider donating the contents.

Top clutter offenders that might exist in various parts of the house include the following:

Magazines. If you have over six month's worth of unread magazines, it's time to consider canceling the subscription and re-subscribing once you have caught up. You could also subscribe to the online edition offered by many print magazines. If you save read magazines, think about the last time you referred to them. I used to save my *Runner's World* magazines. I had three years worth of magazines, but I never went back to reference them. I've since recycled these magazines. Now, I tear out interesting articles that I want to keep instead of the whole magazine. There is so much information available online these days, that even if I throw out an article I decide I want to re-read, I can always look it up at a later date.

Newspapers. I don't know about you, but when I got the daily newspaper, I couldn't keep up with it. It felt like a to-do to read it every day. It typically went straight to the recycle bin without being read. I don't get one anymore. I know many people who can't live without their daily paper. If this is you, by all means, keep getting it (and feel free to skip to the next bullet point). But, if you are like my client, Jill, who had several feet of unread newspapers stacked up, consider making a change. Perhaps you can get your news online or request the printed version on weekends only.

Gifts. Sometimes you get a gift and you just know that you aren't going to use it or you really don't like it. Bypass the clutter stage and immediately put it in the re-gift pile or donate it now. Don't let the gift take up residence in your home.

Some of your discarded items from the cleaning above will head to the trash and some will make it to the recycle bin, but many will still have life left in them and can be a treasure for someone else. Be sure to find a good home for them. It doesn't have to take up a lot of your time. If you think you can sell the item, try selling it on Craigslist or eBay. If it's not something you can sell, think about giving it to a nonprofit organization. Various organizations have regular pickups in our neighborhood, so I have a designated spot in my garage for unwanted items and I put them out on scheduled days. If you don't have this in your neighborhood, oftentimes you can call these organizations and they will do a special pickup.

Another option is to give the items away through Freecycle.org. Freecycle is a grassroots, nonprofit organization that connects people online to give stuff for free in an effort to keep reusable items out of the landfills. They have over nine million members around the world. Membership is free. I have given away many items on Freecycle. I once had a printer that worked haphazardly. I posted it and within two hours I was meeting a mom and her son at a nearby store to give it to them. The best part is, it works both ways. I have benefitted from other people's discards. When I was looking for some *People* magazines for some leisure reading on a trip to Hawaii and some word magnets for a homemade gift I was making for my dad, I posted my request at Freecycle and got what I wanted—for free!

Sometimes I feel like I'm bursting at the seams in a certain part of the house and think that I simply need one more drawer, closet, or room (depending on the severity of the overflow). Whenever this happens, if I take the time to declutter, I find that there are a lot of items I no longer need. It simply takes bringing a fresh perspective to the area and really thinking about whether or not I need the items. Invariably, I find myself with extra room and no need for more space after all.

Although the task of decluttering may seem overwhelming, just do a little at a time. As you go, ask yourself the following three questions to help shed some light on what should stay and what should go.

1. **Have I used it in the past year?** If the answer is no, seriously consider donating it.

2. **What am I keeping this for?** I have a friend who hates to part with anything anyone gave her. If you are like her, can you keep a few of the sentimental items and donate the rest? She also has clothes from decades ago like a red leather dress that she admits she will never wear again. Do you have items like this? If so, why are they still in your closet?

3. **Do I need it?** How much stuff do you really need? Sometimes moving out of accumulation autopilot and bringing a fresh perspective helps us in the decluttering process.

What can you declutter in your physical environment to help declutter your mind?

40

Don't Judge a Weed

If a dandelion weren't classified as a weed, it would probably be seen as a cherished flower or as the nutritious, edible green that it is. When you think about it, dandelions are pretty darn cool. They are believed to have evolved 30 million years ago. They are very unusual looking. They have health benefits. And, lore tells us that if you blow on them, they bring good luck. So, why do they, along with all other weeds, get such a bad rap?

If you look up the definition of a weed, it says, "a plant that is not valued where it is growing and is usually of vigorous growth." I find it interesting that the definition has so much subjectivity to it. Who says that vigorous growth in a yard is a bad thing? For me, a plant that grows without my careful nurturing is my kind of plant. We believe weeds are the enemy because that is what we are taught to believe. What if, instead, we had been taught that having weeds pop up in our yard was a sign of good luck? What if a beautiful yard was the one with the most weeds?

Think about how much time and money you put into killing the weeds in your yard—whether by pulling them individually as they pop up or by spraying them with pesticides (which you then risk bringing into your home). My husband, Dave, reminds me of the character Bill Murray plays in the movie *Caddyshack* but instead of trying to kill the pesky, indestructible gopher, he endlessly battles the clover that invades our lawn. It seems like Dave is working against nature rather than with it in his fight with the clover.

Some people actually promote an all-clover lawn because there are many benefits. It doesn't need to be fertilized, it doesn't suffer the discoloration from dog urine, it aerates the soil on its own, and it stays green all summer long. I'm not saying that I'm ready to have a yard full of weeds just yet, but I do not dislike all weeds simply because they have been classified as such. We should approach weeds with more of an open mind and consider them on an individual basis. As Ralph Waldo Emerson said, *"A weed is a plant whose virtue has not yet been discovered."*

Many weeds are beneficial to our health. Dandelions are packed with minerals such as iron, potassium, beta-carotene, and vitamins A, C, and D. They are also good for cleansing the liver and can help support the digestive system. Stinging nettle, a weed that pops up in the spring, is packed with nutrients. It is a good source of protein and contains high amounts of vitamins A, B, and C, as well as calcium, magnesium, potassium, and zinc. This particular weed is used to help arthritis and allergies, and is often used in detoxification diets. These are just two of many weeds that have health benefits. This is not to say that all weeds are good; it is simply to say that not all weeds are inherently bad.

While I'm plugging weeds, I'd also like to put in a good word for native plants. A native (or indigenous) plant is one that has developed over hundreds or thousands of years in a particular region. They have adapted to the geography and climate of that region. This is in contrast to a non-native plant, which has been introduced by humans. Native plants typically require less fertilizer, water, and care than their non-native counterparts, which is good for you and the environment.

When planning your garden, how about working with nature and finding out which plants are indigenous to your area? And, when you see a weed pop up, rather than immediately reaching for the weed-killer, which is full of toxins, try seeing the weed in a new light. Is it undesirable because you really don't want it growing there or because it has been classified as a weed?

41

Shrinking Your Wasteline

Over an average lifetime, each American will burn 31,350 gallons of gasoline, throw away 128,000 pounds of garbage, and use almost two million gallons of water.[27] It's time for all of us to shed a few pounds of waste.

Using less (energy, plastic, paper) helps to conserve our resources. It reduces green house gases, ground and water pollution, and solid waste. The cleaner our air and fresher our water, the healthier we are. Doing so helps the environment and us. It's a win-win.

Here are eight ideas for reducing waste.

1. **Forgo plastic.** This suggestion is listed first for a reason. It deserves to be starred and highlighted too. Americans throw away millions of plastic bottles every day. I used to buy cases of bottled water. Sure it was convenient to just grab a bottle of water and head out the door. Now I use my reusable bottle. It doesn't take that much extra time, and it is better for the environment and my health. There have been many studies that express concerns about the chemicals in the plastic leaching into the water. This is in addition to the questionable quality of the water that is found in these bottles. An estimated 25% or more of bottled water is really just tap water.[28] Opt instead for a stainless steel or aluminum water bottle, get a filter at home, and fill up.

2. **Carry your own bag.** Carry reusable bags when you shop for clothes, groceries, pet food, and office supplies. I have several reusable bags in the trunk of my car so that they are always with me. At the very least, opt for paper over plastic for bagging. Many plastic bags end up littering the environment and harming wildlife.

3. **Double up the paper.** Printing on both sides of paper is an option for most printers, as is using "fast draft" to save on ink when you don't need best quality. Do this at work, home, and school. We can save on a lot of resources in the manufacturing and recycling of paper if we use less in the first place.

4. **Don't toss the napkins.** When you eat at home, try to get several uses out of your paper napkin. My husband gets about four meals out of each napkin. When you eat out, take only the napkins you need. Cloth napkins are beneficial in that they are reusable, but they have their costs too. Water is used in washing them, energy is used in drying, and there are greenhouse gas emissions in the making of them. The same rule applies, whether you are using paper or cloth: get as many uses out of them as you can.

5. **Let your fingers do the typing.** Now that we have the Internet, phone books have become obsolete in most households. Nonetheless, they still get delivered to us. By calling the number on the inside of the front cover you can request to no longer receive the books. At the very least, these books should be recycled.

6. **Don't flush the meds.** Many people throw old medications in the trash or flush them down the toilet. Neither of these are ideal solutions. Medications thrown in the trash find their way into the soil and those flushed down the toilet make their way into our water supply. According to the U.S. Geological Survey, 80% of waterways tested in the U.S. show traces of common medications such as acetaminophen, hormones, blood pressure medication, codeine, and antibiotics. Studies show these traces of the drugs are impacting aquatic life. Many places like police departments and pharmacies have take-back programs for unwanted medications. Go online to Earth911.com or DisposeMyMeds.org and simply type in your zip code to find a disposal place near you. The same places that take your medications should also accept your unwanted vitamins.

7. **Recycle right.** Check your recycle bin and see if there is any information on it about what is recyclable. Oftentimes, there is a sticker clearly outlining what items are allowed. If that doesn't work, contact your waste company or look on their website. Every time you go to throw an item away, be mindful of where it belongs—trash or recycle bin. If everyone in the U.S. separated the paper, plastic, glass, and aluminum products from the trash and instead put them in the recycle bin, the waste in landfills would be significantly reduced.

8. **Save water.** There are many ways to save water such as watering your lawn deeply (instead of daily) and in the early morning. Watering the lawn early in the day gives the soil and plant roots time to absorb the water without it being evaporated by the sun. Replacing your lawn with

draught-tolerant plants will save even more water. Reusing water from cooking spaghetti or boiling potatoes allows you to feed your plants. Washing your car at a carwash rather than in your driveway is beneficial because the water is recycled and the special draining system prevents pollutants from soap and car grease from entering the groundwater supply.

There are so many ways we can reduce our impact on the environment. I haven't even touched on using LED (light-emitting diode) bulbs instead of incandescent, leaving behind the plastic wrap at the dry cleaners, stopping junk mail, buying Energy Star appliances, and bringing a mug to your favorite coffee shop. It's not about trying to make all of the changes at once; it's about making a few changes at a time. Once those changes become a way of life for you, you can consider taking on a few more.

Many of the chemicals released by landfills and incinerators (where our waste goes) are linked to health concerns like asthma and cancer. The less trash we put in our landfills, the better for our health on many levels.

What changes can you make to shed a few pounds of waste?

42

Frying the Birds

Imagine this. You are at the beach, enjoying the sunny day. You love hearing the waves crashing on the shore and feeling the sand beneath your feet. You are hanging out with good friends wiling away the day. You just finished a delicious picnic. You are in good spirits and decide to commune with nature by sharing some of your leftover French fries with the seagulls nearby. They seem so happy eating the fries just like you were. Ah... life is good.

Life may be good for you in this scenario, but it's not good for the seagull. You may have been well-intentioned in sharing your fries with the birds, but it's harmful for their health. Unfortunately, this happens all too often—at parks, beaches, and restaurants. Birds, squirrels, chipmunks, fish, and sea lions are fed chips, cookies, bread, fries, sandwiches, and more. These foods are not a regular part of a wild animal's diet and can cause significant health problems, including death.

Harm to wildlife comes not only by eating the actual unhealthy food. When animals become dependent on us for their food, their normal migration patterns are interrupted. This can result in them staying too long in an environment that will not support them through the winter or can lead to overpopulation which leads to starvation. It can also become a nuisance where the animals become aggressive because they have become accustomed to getting food from humans.

In addition to not feeding wildlife, it is best to not touch them. I have a friend who touched an endangered sea turtle in Hawaii for his own amusement, despite the fact that he knew it was against the law. Some people even go so far as to try to ride the turtles. The law is set up to protect the turtles from human harassment. It also benefits us because the more we bother the turtles, the less likely they are to feel comfortable being around us. This impacts our being able to see them in their natural habitat.

Being in and appreciating nature brings us health benefits by expanding our worldview and increasing our connectedness to the world around us. This can improve our mood and reduce stress. In most cases, people are not intentionally abusing the wildlife; they are simply self-focused. Next time you encounter wildlife, try to be mindful of doing what's best for them, not you.

Although I've always respected wildlife, my friend, Suzanne, takes it to a whole other level. She protects all creatures—great and small. When Suzanne is out on her morning run during the rainy season, she stops to save every worm that is on the path. She picks them up with a stick and moves them to safety, out of harm's way from walkers, runners, and cyclists. When she swims in her pool, she does her first warm up lap scanning the pool for any bees, flies, spiders, or grasshoppers that need a little boost out of the water. She even moves them to a shaded area so they don't overheat in the sun while trying to recover from their swimming ordeal.

When we expand our compassion circle to include all living creatures, we are less likely to act from a self-focused place and more likely to act in the best interest of the fellow life we've encountered.

It's important to remember that we should be living in a reciprocal relationship with nature. Hurting the wildlife hurts us. Birds are beneficial to us in many ways. They save trees by eating tree-boring insects, protect our lawns by eating grubs and other lawn destroying insects, eat weeds giving us less to battle, keep down the rodent population, and help pollinate our food crops. Insects may seem too small to be of any worth, but they also help us. They pollinate, act as great decomposers to continue the circle of life, and produce useful substances such as wax, honey, and silk.

Next time you encounter wildlife, will you include them in your compassion circle and do what is best for them (and therefore you)?

43

Vinegar and Soda, Please

Imagine that you just cleaned your home and you decide to sit down and relax, appreciating all of your hard work. Suddenly you feel dizzy and are having trouble breathing. Believe it or not, the toxins released from your cleaning products could be the culprit. Even though your house is clean on the surface, toxins abound in the air, and they could be making you sick.

Au Natural in Part Two, the Body quadrant, highlighted the importance of being mindful of the beauty products you use on your skin. This chapter expresses the need to be just as careful with the products you use to clean your home. Many conventional cleaning products harm your health because of the petrochemical VOCs (volatile organic compounds) and synthetic fragrances. The toxins accumulate with each cleaning. They can get into your body through skin contact or inhaling the vapors. Cleaning products can cause dizziness, watery eyes, skin rashes, respiratory problems, and immune system issues. In the long term or in very high exposure, many of these chemicals have been linked to nervous system damage, hormone disruption, and cancer.[29]

Below are a few of the top ingredients to avoid when choosing your cleaning products. Check the labels before you buy.

1. **Petroleum distillates.** Petroleum distillates are found in kitchen and furniture cleaners, and are derived from crude oil sources. They can cause damage to the nervous system and lungs.

2. **Phosphates.** Phosphates are found in some dishwashing detergents. They can increase algae growth in waterways, reducing oxygen sources for aquatic life and decreasing the overall quality of the water. Many states in the U.S. have banned dishwashing detergents with phosphates.

3. **Triclosan.** Triclosan is found in antibacterial products and is believed to disrupt thyroid function.

4. **Ammonia.** Ammonia used to be a common ingredient in glass cleaners, though many companies have stopped using it because it was found to be an eye and lung irritant.

5. **Other** substances to avoid include **chlorine, glycol ethers, phthalates,** and **butyl cellosolve.**

Fortunately, there are many non-toxic cleaning products you can buy in the store. Read the labels and avoid the ingredients above. If you want to save some money and be sure you are using healthy products to clean your house, buy some distilled white vinegar and baking soda. These two products will meet most of your cleaning needs. I like the idea of using products to clean my home that are safe enough for me to ingest. I don't have to worry about compromising my own health or the health of those that might be more susceptible, like pets, children, and aging parents, when I use non-toxic products.

Here are a few ways to use vinegar and baking soda for cleaning.

Vinegar
• Vinegar can be used as a disinfectant, deodorant, and

cleanser for many surfaces such as tile floors, sinks, countertops, mirrors, windows, and appliances. Buy an empty spray bottle and fill it with equal parts water and distilled white vinegar. (Diluting the vinegar with water is advisable to cut the acidity).

- Use it in the laundry as a fabric softener, though do not add it if you are also using chlorine bleach (which is best avoided, altogether) as the fumes created by mixing vinegar with chlorine bleach can be dangerous. I use vinegar when I'm washing my athletic clothes to help remove the odor from technical fabrics because those smells are harder to get out.
- Use it for removing sticky residue, such as those hard-to-remove price labels. (Olive oil works too.) It can also be used to clean the residue that is sometimes left when cleaning with baking soda.

Note: Don't use vinegar on marble, travertine, or limestone. Also, pure vinegar can be too hard on tile grout so be sure to use a diluted solution when cleaning tile floors or counters.

Baking Soda
- Baking soda can be used to remove odors, soften water, dissolve dirt and grime, scrub soap scum, and unclog drains.
- Use it when you need something a little more abrasive than vinegar, like on sinks, toilets, tubs, grout, and counters. You can mix it with water (and lemon) to make a cleansing paste.
- Put an open box in the refrigerator to absorb odors.
- Use it in the laundry for cleaning and as a fabric softener, but add it with the clothes rather than in the fabric softener dispenser where you put the vinegar.
- Use baking soda to remove marks from painted walls by putting a small amount of it on a damp sponge.

Vinegar and Soda

- These two natural cleaning agents combine well for bigger jobs. There will be a little fizz when you combine the two. You can use these two in combination to get stains out of carpets and clothes. Sprinkle on some baking soda, then spray on vinegar. Scrub and let the surface dry. The excess can be vacuumed out of carpets when dry or washed out of clothes as you would normally. (It's always best to do a spot test first.)

- Vinegar and soda also work well together to unclog drains. Pour a cup of baking soda into the drain, followed by a cup of vinegar. Wait several minutes, and then flush the drain with hot water. If this doesn't work, a plumber's snake is also a good alternative to the harsher, extremely toxic concoctions that you buy in the store.

Because we have so many choices when we go to the store, we get caught up in the complexity of it all. Aisles are lined with an overwhelming number of cleaning products for every imaginable purpose. Try to go back to the basics. It is safer for your health and for the environment, and it will save you money too.

Next time you are at the store looking for cleaning products, will you ask the salesperson for vinegar and soda, please?

44

No More Litter Bugs

The other day I was in the car waiting for my husband to get some items at the grocery store and I saw a man come out of the store with a pack of cigarettes. He opened the pack on the way to his car, throwing the wrapper on the ground. This is not an isolated incident. Within the same week, I saw a woman carrying her Starbucks coffee, and granted, she did have her hands full, but she dropped her napkin. She saw it fall behind her and walked on. Why do people feel entitled to litter?

Over 51 billion pieces of litter land on U.S. roadways each year. On roadways, cigarette butts are the most littered item, followed by paper, and then plastic. Off roadways, mostly at entrances to businesses and transportation, the top littered items are candy wrappers and cigarette butts. People litter for a variety of reasons: they don't care, litter begets litter, ignorance, lack of pride, and lack of consequence for their actions. When we litter, we have a very limited view of the world around us.

As we are discovering throughout the Environment section, everything that happens in and to the environment happens to us. Littering is no different. When we litter, we harm the environment and we harm ourselves, as highlighted below:[30]

- **Reduces property values.** Houses for sale in neighborhoods with litter problems are valued lower, estimated at a seven percent decrease in property value.
- **Starts fires.** Fires started by litter cause millions of dollars of damages every year.

- **Causes car accidents.** Every year there are numerous car accidents caused by attempting to avoid litter in the roadways.
- **Kills wildlife.** Millions of birds, fish, and animals die annually from eating, trying to digest, or getting trapped in litter.
- **Promotes the spread of germs.** Litter carries germs.
- **Costs money.** Litter costs money. Litter cleanup costs the U.S. almost 11.5 billion dollars each year.

Here are four steps you can take to help reduce litter:

1. **Plan ahead.** When you go for a hike or to a park, plan ahead by bringing an extra bag to pick up any litter you find along the way. Better yet, leave a bag in your car for anytime you find litter and can't find a place to dispose of it.

2. **Make it fun.** You can make it a game for the family on who can find the most litter. Have the kids simply point out the trash for you to pick up so that they don't touch it.

3. **Educate others.** If you see a friend or family member littering, politely educate them about the consequences of their actions. If you see someone you don't know doing it, consider pointing it out if you feel you can do so without confrontation. Otherwise, pick it up yourself and take comfort in knowing that you did a good deed.

4. **Volunteer.** Join an organization like Keep America Beautiful or find a local Adopt-A-Road program through your state's environment departments. Spend a day with likeminded individuals cleaning up the environment.

The rewards for caring for the environment are numerous and can carry over into all four quadrants. You can get exercise (Body), feel good about yourself (Mind), connect with others (Relationships), and be out in nature (Environment).

What steps can you take to help keep your environment litter-free?

45

Stop the (Holiday) Madness

I'm not a holiday grinch, but I cringe at the waste that comes from the holiday season every year. From Thanksgiving to New Years Day, household waste in the U.S. increases by more than 25%.[31] This holiday season, think about giving a gift to the environment by reducing waste. In doing so, you'll be giving a gift to yourself as well—less stress, less mess, fewer dollars spent, and more time for fun!

Even though this time period is only one-twelfth of the year, the waste generated warrants an entire chapter dedicated to it. Think about the amount of trash piled high with food, holiday cards, ribbon, paper, and packaging—much of which is not recyclable. This adds up to an additional one million tons a week to our landfills during this time.[32] The waste then sits in landfill for hundreds of years before it decomposes. This isn't healthy for the environment or for us. Start planning ahead for the upcoming holiday season and see if you can commit to trying any of the eight ideas below.

1. **Limit the holiday cards.** Did you know that the 2.65 billion holiday cards sold each year in the U.S. could fill a football field 10 stories high? If we each send one card less, we'd save 50,000 cubic yards of paper.[33] How about sending electronic cards or posting a holiday video for your friends on YouTube? Last year, I was sent an e-card from a friend through St. Jude Children's Research Hospital. What a lovely

idea to make a donation in honor of your friends and family and support such a worthy cause at the same time. For paper or photo cards, think about only sending to those friends and family who are out-of-town that you don't see as often. This will save you both time and money. I stopped sending holiday cards a few years ago and I don't miss that extra to-do around the holidays.

2. **Go potted or rent.** Each year 50 million Christmas trees are purchased in the U.S., and of those, about 30 million go to landfill.[34] Artificial trees can be reused, but are not ideal for the environment either. They are made of PVC (a harmful plastic), are typically shipped from outside the U.S. (consuming resources to get to their final destination), and are not recyclable or biodegradable. Instead, go for a potted tree that can be replanted after the holiday season. If you don't want to plant it in your yard, you can find another spot for it. The Original Christmas Tree Company has some ideas. There are also companies that rent trees, such as Rent a Living Christmas Tree. Both of these companies can be found online.

3. **Try homemade.** Give homemade gifts instead of packaged ones. The sentiment will last a lifetime. At my dad's house, we now give homemade gifts instead of purchased ones. We have done this for the past four years. We draw names and make a gift for one person. I cherish the photo calendar my dad made me, the painted box with uplifting sayings my sister made me, the wood-carved wine holder my brother-in-law made me, and the decorated frames my stepmom gave me. I may not remember all of the store-bought gifts I have received from them over the years, but I

will always remember the homemade ones.

4. **Give less.** If you are not ready to give up gift giving entirely, how about drawing names and simply buying for one person? This means less time in the mall and lower January credit card bills. For less packaging waste, good gift ideas are movie tickets, spa certificates, gift cards, or vouchers for an activity shared together. My friend, Bev, exchanges the "gift of time" with her friends whereby they commit to doing a social activity together in the New Year. Over the years, she has enjoyed museum visits, concerts, and walking tours with her friends. Another great idea is to make a donation to an organization that has meaning for the person you are gifting.

   For me, it's not only about the money—it's about the time and pressure of gift giving. The holiday frenzy is only exacerbated by the obligation of gift giving. Give yourself a chance to enjoy the season without putting so many demands on your time (and pocketbook).

5. **Create traditions.** Some of my favorite holiday traditions are building ginger bread houses, eating fondue, cooking potato pancakes, building puzzles, playing games, and driving through the neighborhood listening to holiday music and seeing the decorative lights. Creating traditions that your family looks forward to puts less emphasis on gift giving and more emphasis on quality family time.

6. **Be creative with gift wrap.** Try using newspapers, magazines, old calendars, or scarves to wrap presents. Choose wrapping paper with recycled content. Don't throw out the scraps. Use them and wrap a gift with several scrap pieces.

Go light (or not at all) on the tissue paper. Instead of throwing out (or recycling) all of the tissue paper, boxes, and gift wrap, save it for next year. My sister, Debbie, and her husband, Vince, outdid themselves last year when they wrapped my gifts in fresh banana leaves that could be returned to nature after I opened my gifts because they know how important being kind to the environment is to me.

7. **Forgo the ribbons and bows.** If every family reused just two feet of holiday ribbon, the 38,000 miles of ribbon saved could tie a bow around the entire planet.[35] It's the gift inside that matters, not the packaging.

8. **Save energy.** I enjoy the holiday lights as much as the next person but they use a lot of energy. If you are in the market for new lights, buy LED ones. They save energy. If you are using older lights, add a timer to make sure they turn off after midnight to save energy.

Okay, so maybe I am a bit of a holiday grinch—limited holiday cards, rented Christmas trees, and homemade gifts? I've made most of these changes over the years, and I have to say—the holidays are much less stressful (and more meaningful) for me than they used to be. I have time to enjoy the season and my family. I'm not running around like a crazy person making sure I have gifts for everyone, holiday cards filled out, and gifts wrapped. It's liberating.

On the other hand, I do enjoy getting into the holiday spirit by listening to the holiday music, seeing the lights, and receiving the photo cards and witty letters from my friends. Four Quadrant Living is not about depriving ourselves of the things that bring us pleasure. Pleasure is a key component of our health. If there are certain items listed above that bring you joy during the holiday season, by all means, do them. Just do them mindfully, recognizing the impact on the health of the environment, those around you, and even yourself.

You don't have to make all of the changes, but are there one or two that you can make for the next holiday season as a gift to the environment, as well as to yourself?

46

Sleep Deprivation Unit

When my sister was in the hospital for three weeks undergoing stem cell transplant, my family and I took shifts spending the days and nights with her so that she was never alone. We used to joke that the hospital was a "sleep deprivation unit" because there was definitely no rest for the weary. Lights were bright, noises abounded, and nurse visits were frequent. We think of a hospital as a place to heal, but the environment is not very conducive to this.

Hospitals typically have a sterile and impersonal atmosphere. There is no connection to the outside. There are few windows, so almost no sunshine gets in. There is no fresh air, with the recycled air just circling around and around. All too often, unappetizing and unhealthy food is served at hospitals—food that is low in nutrients and fiber, and high in pesticides, preservatives, trans fats, and high fructose corn sugar. In fact, one study showed that 59 percent of children's hospitals researched had fast-food restaurants on site.[36]

Instead of the typical hospital environment, imagine a place that looked like this instead:

- Volunteers at hospital entrance welcoming visitors.
- Serene landscapes with trees, flowers, and water features for patients and guests to enjoy. Views from most rooms, hallways, and waiting areas.

- Single occupancy in all rooms and doors that open to garden settings.

- Colorful, happy art hanging in patient rooms.

- Music systems in addition to televisions.

- Fresh, local, healthy food served.

- Noise reduction through less overhead paging.

- Windows and skylights so patients and staff can stay in sync with the sun.

- Windows open to allow in fresh air during day. HEPA filters circulate air at night.

- No limits on the number of visitors and no designated visiting hours. Sleep chairs or extra beds available for guests.

- Walls and floors designed in warm colors.

- Wide hallways for a sense of space.

- Power cables buried deeper than required by code to reduce harmful effects of electric and magnetic fields.

- Special water filtration systems for clean water.

- Health-friendly construction materials used to build the hospital and non-toxic products used for cleaning.

- Complementary healing modalities available including acupuncture, chiropractic, naturopathy, massage therapy, guided imagery, and healing touch.

- Patients able to bring their own herbal remedies to use with permission from their doctors.

- Dogs brought in as part of a pet therapy program to cheer up patients.

Doesn't it seem like this environment with serene landscapes, nutritious food, reduced noise, and pet therapy would be more conducive to healing than what we typically find in hospitals? You may be thinking that this list is a bit far-fetched and I'm living in fantasyland, but, guess what? This hospital actually exists. It is the North Hawaii Community Hospital and was built around the idea that body, mind, spirit, culture, nature, and community are all important in the healing process. It is designed around patient-centered care.

There have been studies that support how these environmental elements aid in the healing process. One study showed that patients who had a view of nature instead of a brick wall needed less pain medication, suffered fewer minor complications (such as fever, nausea, and constipation), and stayed less time at the hospital.[37] Another study showed that post-op patients who recovered in sunny rooms needed 20% less pain medication per hour than patients in darker rooms.[38]

Hospitals are businesses, so we can't expect them to make changes unless it makes economic sense. With North Hawaii Community Hospital and other patient-centered healing centers leading the way, hopefully businesses will be able to see that there is a way to do the right thing *and* make a profit at the same time.

Even though you will be spending less time in the hospital if you are engaging in Four Quadrant Living, there may be times when we, or our loved ones, need to be there. Until all hospitals are designed as healing centers, we can make our own small changes in this environment to help the healing process. Here are five ideas.

1. **Play the tunes.** Bring in an iPod and a headset so your loved one can play music that makes her feel happy and calm.

2. **Feel the love.** Place pictures of friends and family around the room to help her feel supported and connected to others even when they aren't there.

3. **Bring the outdoors in.** If the room doesn't have a window, display some nature photos to help bring in the outdoors.

4. **Set the mood.** Drape a few scarves around the room to add some warmth and color.

5. **Nourish the body.** After checking first with the doctor for any food restrictions, bring in some fresh, healthy, and appetizing food so that your loved one is properly nourished.

Next time you, or a family member, are in the hospital, what small changes can you make to create more of a peaceful, relaxing environment and less of a stressful, sleep-deprivation unit?

47

Eating for the Planet

Do you know where your food comes from, how it was produced, and what it took to get to you? Every time you purchase and consume food, you are implicitly supporting its hidden history. This history includes geography (local or international), production methods (organic or conventional, and natural or genetically modified), and economic system (fair or free trade). Eating for the planet is about making more informed and conscious nutrition decisions.

In Part Two, the Body quadrant, we talked about eating well for our own health. This chapter gives nine ideas for taking healthy eating one step further by eating well for ourselves *and* for the environment.

1. **Go local.** As mentioned earlier, food typically travels 1,500 miles to reach our plates, depleting nutrients along the way. When you eat local, you support your local economy and reduce carbon emissions. Local food is picked when it is ripe and is much fresher when you eat it. Today you could be eating an egg that was laid yesterday or strawberries that were picked today. For local food, try shopping at farmers markets or join a CSA (Community Supported Agriculture). CSA foods are seasonally grown, requiring fewer pesticides and fertilizers since they are grown at optimum times during the year. Check out LocalHarvest.org to find a CSA near you.

2. **Buy organic.** Conventional foods are sprayed with pesticides and fertilizers, which isn't good for the earth, the farmers, or your family. These chemical pollutants get into our soil, waterways, and air. Many of the herbicides and insecticides that we use widely in the U.S. are banned in Europe and other countries because of health concerns. Buy organic, especially when purchasing those fruits and vegetables that are high in pesticides. See *Fad-Free Eating* in Part Two, the Body quadrant, for a list of which produce to buy organic.

3. **Eat it all.** Next time you are eating a fruit or vegetable, think about using all parts of it—including celery tops, orange peels, and beet greens. The leaves of broccoli (one ounce) provide 90% of daily vitamin A requirement while the florets only deliver three percent. Orange peels contain more than four times as much fiber as the fruit inside. You can grate them and put them on vegetables such as green beans or asparagus. Use Swiss chard stems for soups. Try sautéing beet greens with lemon and garlic. Use vegetable ends to make broth. Save waste and get some great nutrients by eating it all.

4. **Load up on plants.** Eating a diet heavy on foods from plants—fruits and vegetables (organic for those with high pesticides) and whole grains (non-GMO)—is good for you and for the environment. The farming of cattle requires significant energy and pollutes the earth. It takes a lot of resources (water, land, and food) to raise a cow, which can feed much fewer people than the resources used for growing vegetables. If you eat meat, eat less of it. See meat as an accent to your food rather than having it front and center in such large portions. To ensure the animals have been treated humanely, look for meat labeled Certified Humane

Raised and Handled, Animal Welfare Approved, or American Humane Certified.

5. **Skip the process.** Leave the processed foods on the shelves and opt instead for whole foods like fruit, vegetables, and whole grains. Processed foods use a lot of packaging which ends up in our landfills. Instead of reaching for potato chips, buy the whole potato instead. There will be no bag to throw out when you are done.

6. **Support green business.** Buy from those companies that are making an effort to use less packaging, use recycled content in their packaging, purchase their supplies from local companies, and use organic ingredients.

7. **Grow your own.** When you eat, do you think about how the food got from the soil to your plate? By growing your own, you will have a better understanding of the food cycle, from seedling to edible product. This is a fun project for the whole family.

8. **Compost.** Composting is a great way to turn your yard and food waste into healthy nutrients for your garden, and keeps this waste out of landfills.

9. **Be thankful.** If you don't grow your own, be thankful for the farmers who planted and tended to the food. Appreciate the sun and soil that made the food grow. Be grateful for the many people who transported the food so it got to your plate. Understanding the source of the food we eat brings mindfulness to our eating and helps us to make better choices.

The basic laws of economics tell us about supply and demand. We can affect change by demanding food that is healthy for us and for the environment. The supply will follow our demand.

When you purchase your next week's groceries, can you make a few changes that are best for you *and* the planet?

48

My Love Affair with a Mountain

My love affair with a mountain began almost 15 years ago when I first moved to the East Bay of San Francisco. As soon as I laid eyes on the 3,849-foot beauty that is Mount Diablo, I knew it was love at first sight. Since that time, I have enjoyed numerous hikes, runs, strolls, and picnics on the mountain. I love watching the colors of the mountain change throughout the year—from lush green in the winter to golden brown in the summer. I enjoy spending time on the mountain alone as well as with friends. I feel lighter and more at peace when I am on the mountain.

Many think that nature is a "nice to have," but it is actually a "must have" if we are to live in a sustainable environment. Fifty percent of the increased carbon in the air is from land that has been converted from open space to developed areas and agriculture. Mount Diablo and all other open spaces are helping to save the planet by reducing the carbon footprint and by producing oxygen. The amount of carbon that is stored in a park the size of Mount Diablo is the equivalent of removing over 16,000 passenger cars from the road annually! Parklands the size of Mount Diablo produce approximately 66,000 metric tons of oxygen annually.[39] There are many open spaces around the world, like Mount Diablo, that are helping to save our planet. Unfortunately many of these lands are threatened by mining opportunities, lack of funding, and land development.

Mount Diablo is only one of my many natural loves. When I think of times where I have felt connected to something larger than myself, nature is always involved. I felt it while watching sea turtles at night in Costa Rica travel one hundred yards up the shore to lay their softball size eggs. I felt it while sitting on the mountaintop in the Canadian Rockies once I had climbed to the top and looked out at the open expanse. I felt it in Antarctica and not hearing or seeing any sounds or structures made by humans. I marvel at nature's true awesomeness.

Nature gives us so much. It gives us beautiful places to explore, clean air to breathe, solace and serenity from its beauty, culture and history to connect us to our past, an opportunity to see wildlife in its natural habitat, and a connection to something larger than ourselves. The more we appreciate nature in all of its splendid glory, the more living green will become a part of our daily lives. Once we learn to see that nature can give us health, we will do what we can to protect it.

Nature connects and unites us all. It exists all over the world and the feeling we get from it is universal—transcending religion, economics, gender, and politics. What are the times in your life when you saw the bigger picture and felt wonder because of what you saw? What spots near and far have touched your heart? What do you hear and see? What other humans, animals, and plants share it with you? What history do you know about your spot and what is there still to learn about it? How do you feel when you are there?

This week, get out into nature and experience it in all of its grandeur. Thank it for the health that it gives to you and to the rest of us. Vow to take care of it as well as you take care of yourself.

Is Your Environment Healthy?

Indicators for health and illness in the Environment quadrant focus on the health of our environment. Toxins in our environment and our connectedness to the world can affect our health. A "yes" answer represents an indicator for health and a "no" for illness, unless otherwise noted.

- Do you have access to organically and locally grown food?
- Does the city you live in have good air quality?
- Do you have access to clean drinking water?
- Do you take part in environmental activities, such as recycling?
- Do you have access to natural settings near your work or home?
- Do you actively work to reduce waste?
- Do you spend time in nature?
- Do you use non-toxic cleaning products?
- Do you eat with the planet in mind?
- Are you aware of the impact your actions have on others and the world around you?
- Do you feel engaged with the world?
- Do you have moments of silence?
- Do you live and work in a clean, litter-free environment?
- Do you feel safe?
- Do you use pesticides in your garden? ("yes" is illness indicator)
- Is your home or work space cluttered? ("yes" is illness indicator)

- Do you live near a toxic waste site? ("yes" is illness indicator)

Guided by the ideas in this section, look at where you answered "no" in the earlier questions and try to identify how these can become "yes." Do the same for the last three questions if you answered "yes" and try to figure out how they can become "no."

EPILOGUE

Congratulations! By reading this book, you have taken the first step in making healthy living your new way of life. You are on your way to creating your new health destiny!

If you have already tried a few ideas in the book, that's fantastic. If you haven't yet made any changes, what are you waiting for? It may take time to change your body, but it takes a split second to change your mind. You can decide right now to get on the path to a healthier you. Don't wait for your wake-up call. Value your health before sickness comes. Be proactive now.

Although we have looked at each quadrant separately, the four quadrants are intimately interconnected. They do not operate in isolation. A change in one quadrant affects the others. You are not just your body, mind, relationships, or environment. In any given moment, you are all of them.

Recognizing the dynamic interplay of the quadrants empowers us. If something feels out of our control in one quadrant, we can focus on a different quadrant that feels in our control, thus promoting better overall health. Mindfully recognizing this allows us to prevent the domino effect of illness overwhelming us.

You don't have to adopt every idea and practice in the book. Begin by finding one or two ideas from each of the four quadrants that resonate most with you and try them out. After a few weeks, you can take on a few more. Set yourself up for success by starting where you are at, not where you want to or think you should be.

Pleasure is a key component of health, so stressing about what you are eating and how often you are exercising could counteract your new health practices. Having fun with Four Quadrant Living is the key to making healthy living a part of who you are, rather than something you do.

People often think that living healthy means sacrifice, but when healthy living comes from within—from your values, beliefs, and vision you have for yourself—eating well and making lifestyle changes doesn't feel like a sacrifice. It feels like a privilege, an active choice, and simply your new way of life.

I hope the ideas in this book inspire you to expect more from life than to just survive. It is your time to thrive and live radiantly—to live with abundant health, vitality, and happiness.

A NOD TO INTEGRAL THEORY AND EPIGENETICS

In the introduction, I said that two untruths had inspired this book. The first untruth, that health comes from treating only the Body, is discredited by all of the research supporting a four quadrant model. Taking into account the Mind, Relationships, and Environment is also essential for our understanding and treatment of health and disease.

Looking at health in a four quadrant context is inspired by Ken Wilber's Integral Theory. Ken Wilber, author of over 20 books and founder of the Integral Institute, is a visionary and philosopher of science and society. He promotes Integral Theory, a comprehensive world philosophy, as a way to understand human life and potential. He uses the term "integral" to mean all-inclusive. This theory provides a map of the whole picture and can be used in business, medicine, law, ecology, politics, and education. It is based on a four quadrant model. Ken Wilber's four quadrants are I, It, We, and Its. (The four quadrant model is one of five elements of Integral Theory. The other elements are beyond the scope of this book.)

Four Quadrant Living takes Integral Theory and applies it to health, as shown in the figure below.

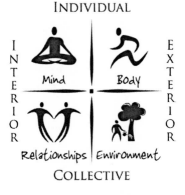

The quadrants represent the interior and exterior as well as the individual and collective aspects of our lives. The top two quadrants, Mind and Body, represent the individual. The bottom two quadrants, Relationships and Environment, represent the collective. The left two quadrants, Mind and Relationships, represent the interior while the right two, Body and Environment, reflect the exterior.

Mind (I) = Interior Individual
Body (It) = Exterior Individual
Relationships (We) = Interior Collective
Environment (Its) = Exterior Collective

Each quadrant interacts with and influences the others. The individual affects the collective and vice versa; likewise, the interior impacts the exterior and vice versa. For example, our individual health is impacted by the health of others, our relationships, and the environment. We may be eating well and exercising, but we cannot truly be healthy if at the same time our mind is stressed, our relationships are toxic, and our world is sick. Similarly, our relationships will suffer if we do not tend to our mental and emotional well-being.

The second untruth, that we are our genes, is refuted by the science of epigenetics, which is regulating gene expression without altering DNA. This science is the foundation of why this book matters, because how we live our life *does* impact our health. I first learned about epigenetics when I read Bruce Lipton's *The Biology of Belief.* This book changed my life. It talks about how research in the field of cell biology and quantum physics is showing that genes and DNA do not totally control our biology. Our genes are influenced by signals outside our cells by such factors as nutrition, stress, lifestyle, and emotions.

In the 1980s, the Human Genome project, an effort led by an international group of scientists, was designed to understand the genetic code of life by sequencing the human chromosomes. The outcome was the discovery that our genetic structure is not as rigid as originally thought. It is now recognized that our *genotype*—our genetic makeup—gets transformed into our *phenotype* as a result of nutritional, lifestyle, and environmental influences. Our health is determined not by our genotype, but rather by our phenotype, the combination of our genetics and environment.

I thank Ken Wilber and Bruce Lipton for opening my mind to new ways of seeing health. Ken Wilber's Integral Theory gave me the context of seeing a whole view of health—Mind, Body, Relationships, and Environment—and inspiring me to come up with the name for my company and book, "Four Quadrant Living." Bruce Lipton provided the foundation for why living this way matters—because how we live our life *does* impact our health.

ACKNOWLEDGEMENTS

I will will always be grateful to Fall Ferguson for saying "yes" because it was the impetus I needed to start writing this book. Thank you to my editor, B. Lynn Goodwin. I appreciate your fast turnaround and helpful comments. Hiring Roger C. Parker as my coach in the 11th hour was the best thing I could have done. You were truly my lifeline for maintaining my sanity and moving the project forward.

Thank you to my clients for trusting me on your journey to a healthier you. It has been an honor and inspiration to work with you. A special thank you to the clients mentioned in this book for allowing me to share your stories so that others could learn from them. Although I have permission from everyone, I have changed names and other details to help protect their identities.

Thank you to Four Quadrant Living supporters around the world who have connected via social media. It has been fun, enlightening, and motivating to share ideas with you about healthy living.

Thank you to Linda Clark, my teacher and mentor. Because of you, I have a deep understanding of the connection between health and nutrition. Thank you to Janet Fazio, my graphic and web designer, for supporting me in the beginning stages and helping me build my brand. Thank you to Jenny B. Jones and Cynthia Ruzzi for being early editors of this book. Your insights and comments helped me to take a step back and make the book even better.

Thank you to all of my friends and family who have supported me along the way. I want to especially thank Tracy Achelis, Kathie Taylor, and Aunt Joan Gordon for being big supporters of Four

Quadrant Living, helping me keep the faith that the message I am trying to share has value and is important. I am grateful to my friends Rachelle Fong, Liz Lyons, and Beth Morin for always giving me the encouragement I needed when I had my doubts. A special acknowledgement goes to Tiffany Deusebio for being my "CMO" and Varsha Khatri for being my weekly accountability buddy; also, to Bev Benzon and Christy Slye not only for editing the book but also for being my reliable and wise sounding board.

Thank you to my dad and stepmom, David and Diane Colman. Diane, thank you for always believing that I can do anything I set my mind to. Dad, it meant a lot (especially coming from a retired physician), when you sent out a note to all of your friends telling them about my website and how you believed in the message. Thank you to my mom, Diane Colman, for always being so supportive and proud of me, and for encouraging me to continually "reinvent" myself. I am now officially an author.

Thank you to my sister, Debbie Colman, my "biggest cheerleader," for always being excited about my accomplishments and sad for my disappointments. You have inspired me by showing the power of the mind in illness. You treated your aggressive cancer with forceful treatment, both physically and mentally. I admire that you truly knew in your heart that when treatment was over, you were cancer-free. Here you are, 15 years later, married to the man of your dreams with a thriving insurance business. You deserve all of the health and happiness life has to offer. "Celebrate good times, come on!"

Finally, a big thank you to my husband, David Luczynski, for always supporting my latest (crazy and lofty) endeavors. You not only support them, you join in them with your mind and heart wide open—like trying sardines when I learned how good they are for us or deciding to run a marathon when we were not runners. You have always believed in me and given me the freedom and encouragement to be true to myself and pursue my passions. Thank you from the bottom of my heart for the many hours you patiently and wholeheartedly spent with me to make this book come to fruition, from beginning to end. I love you and take great comfort in knowing I can count on you, always.

Here is what I know for sure: We are the creators of our own lives. Actively and passionately choose the life you want. Seek out meaning, be happy, appreciate life, live mindfully, be authentic, share the journey with others, and walk softly on this earth.

NOTES

[1] Centers for Disease Control and Prevention, www.cdc.gov; National Cancer Institute, www.cancer.gov

[2] American Heart Association, www.heart.org; American Institute for Cancer Research, www.aicr.org; World Health Organization, www.who.int

[3] Centers for Disease Control and Prevention, www.cdc.gov

[4] The American Institute of Stress, www.stress.org

[5] Blakeslee, S. (1998, October 13). Placebos prove so powerful even experts are surprised: New studies explore the brain's triumph over reality. *New York Times.* Retrieved from www.nytimes.com

[6] Voelker, R. (1996). Nocebos contribute to a host of ills. *Journal of the American Medical Association, 275*(5), 345-47.

[7] Robison, J., & Carrier, K. (2004). *The spirit and science of holistic health: More than broccoli, jogging, and bottled water… more than yoga, herbs, and meditation.* Bloomington, IN: AuthorHouse, p. 95.

[8] Centers for Disease Control and Prevention, www.cdc.gov

[9] Centers for Disease Control and Prevention, www.cdc.gov

[10] Small Plate Movement, www.smallplatemovement.org

[11] National Sleep Foundation, www.sleepfoundation.org

[12] National Sleep Foundation, www.sleepfoundation.org

[13] National Institutes of Health, www.nih.gov

[14] Enig, M., & Fallon, S. (2006). *Eat fat, lose fat: The healthy alternative to trans fats.* New York, NY: Plume.

[15] Non-GMO Project, www.nongmoproject.org

[16] Environmental Working Group, www.ewg.org

[17] Environmental Working Group, www.ewg.org; National Institutes of Health, www.nih.gov

[18] Petersen, M. (2008). *Our daily meds: How the pharmaceutical companies transformed themselves into slick marketing machines and hooked the nation on prescription drugs.* New York, NY: Picador, pp. 6-7.

[19] Goldberg, C. (2013, April 22). National study: Teen misuse and abuse of prescription drugs up 33 percent since 2008, stimulants contributing to sustained Rx epidemic. Retrieved from www.drugfree.org

[20] Saputo, L. (with Belitsos, B.). (2009). *A return to healing: Radical health care reform and the future of medicine.* San Rafael, CA: Origin Press, pp. 114-115.

[21] National Institutes of Health, www.nih.gov

[22] Starfield, B. (2000). Is US health really the best in the world? *Journal American Medical Association, 284*(4), 483-5; Null, G., et al. Death by Medicine, *Nutrition Institute of America.*

[23] The American Society for Aesthetic Plastic Surgery, www.surgery.org

[24] Jourard, S.M. (1966). An exploratory study of body accessibility. *British Journal of Social and Clinical Psychology, 5,* 221-231.

[25] U.S. PIRG, the Federation of State Public Interest Research Groups, www.uspirg.org

[26] Barton, J., & Pretty, J. (2010). What is the best dose of nature and green exercise for improving mental health? A multi-study analysis. *Environmental Science and Technology, 44*(10), 3947-3955.

[27] Carangelo, A., & Grossman, A. (2008). Human footprint, *National Geographic.* Retrieved from www.nationalgeographic.com

[28] Natural Resources Defense Council, www.nrdc.org

[29] United States Environmental Protection Agency, www.epa.gov

[30] Keep America Beautiful, www.kag.org

[31] United States Environmental Protection Agency, www.epa.gov

[32] United States Environmental Protection Agency, www.epa.gov

[33] The Use Less Stuff Report, www.use-less-stuff.com

[34] The Use Less Stuff Report, www.use-less-stuff.com

[35] The Use Less Stuff Report, www.use-less-stuff.com

[36] Sahud, H., et al. (2006). Marketing fast food: Impact of fast food restaurants in children's hospitals. *Pediatrics, 118*(6), 2290-97.

[37] Ulrich, R.S. (1984). View through a window may influence recovery from surgery. *Science, 224*(4), 420-421.

[38] Walch, J.M., et al. (2005). The effect of sunlight on postoperative analgesic medication use: A prospective study of patients undergoing spinal surgery. *Psychosomatic Medicine, 67*, 156–63.

[39] Save Mount Diablo, www.savemountdiablo.org

BIBLIOGRAPHY

Listed below, by section, are the principal works referred to in the text as well as others that supplied me with facts or contributed to my thinking.

General

Buettner, D. (2008). *The blue zones: Lessons for living longer from the people who've lived the longest.* Washington, D.C.: National Geographic Society.

Dacher, E. (2006). *Integral health: The path to human flourishing.* Laguna Beach, CA: Basic Health Publications.

Lipton, B. (2011). *The biology of belief: Unleashing the power of consciousness, matter, & miracles.* Carlsbad, CA: Hay House.

Moustakas, C. (1990). *Heuristic research: Design, methodology, and applications.* Newbury Park, CA: Sage.

Robbins, J. (2006). *Healthy at 100: The scientifically proven secrets of the world's healthiest and longest-lived peoples.* New York, NY: Random House.

Robison, J., & Carrier, K. (2004). *The spirit and science of holistic health: More than broccoli, jogging, and bottled water...more than yoga, herbs, and meditation.* Bloomington, IN: Author-House.

Saputo, L. (with Belitsos, B.). (2009). *A return to healing: Radical health care reform and the future of medicine.* San Rafael, CA: Origin Press.

Wilber, K., Patten, T., Leonard, A., & Morelli, M. (2008). *Integral life practice: A 21st century blueprint for physical health, emotional balance, mental clarity, and spiritual awakening.* Boston, MA: Integral Books.

Wilber, K. (2007). *Integral spirituality: A startling new role for religion in the modern and postmodern world.* Boston, MA: Shambhala.

Wilber, K. (2007). *The integral vision: A very short introduction to the revolutionary integral approach to life, God, the universe, and everything.* Boston, MA: Shambhala.

Part One: Mind

Carlson, R. (1997). *Don't sweat the small stuff...and it's all small stuff: Simple ways to keep the little things from taking over your life.* New York, NY: Hyperion.

Seaward, B.L. (2009). *Managing stress: Principles and strategies for health and well-being.* Sudbury, MA: Jones and Bartlett.

Seaward, B.L. (2008). *The art of peace and relaxation workbook.* Sudbury, MA: Jones and Bartlett.

Tolle, E. (2006). *A new earth: Awakening to your life's purpose.* New York, NY: Penguin.

Tolle, E. (1999). *The power of now: A guide to spiritual enlightenment.* Novato, CA: New World Library.

Part Two: Body

Angell, M. (2005). *The truth about the drug companies: How they deceive us and what to do about it.* New York, NY: Random House.

Bland, J.S. (1999). *Genetic nutritioneering: How you can modify inherited traits and live a longer, healthier life.* Los Angeles, CA: Keats.

Brownlee, S. (2007). *Overtreated: Why too much medicine is making us sicker and poorer.* New York, NY: Bloomsbury.

Enig, M., & Fallon, S. (2006). *Eat fat, lose fat: The healthy alternative to trans fats.* New York, NY: Plume.

Epstein, S., & Fitzgerald, R. (2009). *Toxic beauty: How cosmetics and personal-care products endanger your health…and what you can do about it.* Dallas, TX: BenBella.

Petersen, M. (2008). *Our daily meds: How the pharmaceutical companies transformed themselves into slick marketing machines and hooked the nation on prescription drugs.* New York, NY: Picador.

Pollan, M. (2009). *Food rules: An eater's manual.* New York, NY: Penguin.

Pollan, M. (2008). *In defense of food: An eater's manifesto.* New York, NY: Penguin.

Taubes, G. (2008). *Good calories, bad calories: Fats, carbs, and the controversial science of diet and health.* New York, NY: Anchor.

Williams, R.J. (1998). *Biochemical individuality: The key to understanding what shapes your health.* New Canaan, CT: Keats.

Part Three: Relationships

Bennet-Goleman, T. (2001). *Emotional alchemy: How the mind can heal the heart.* New York, NY: Three Rivers Press.

Ornish, D. (1998). *Love and survival: 8 pathways to intimacy and health.* New York, NY: HarperCollins.

Pavuk, P., & Pavuk, S. (2000). *The story of a lifetime: A keepsake of personal memoirs.* Santa Fe, NM: TriAngel.

Pert, C. (1999). *Molecules of emotion: The science behind mind-body medicine.* New York, NY: Touchstone.

Sose, B. (1991). *Talk to me.* Winter Park, FL: Character Builders.

Stock, G. (1987). *The book of questions.* New York, NY: Workman Publishing.

Part Four: Environment

Riebel, L. (2011). *The green foodprint: Food choices for healthy people and a healthy planet.* Lafayette, CA: Print and Pixel.

Rogers, E., & Kostigen, T.M. (2007). *The green book: The everyday guide to saving the planet one simple step at a time.* New York, NY: Three Rivers Press.

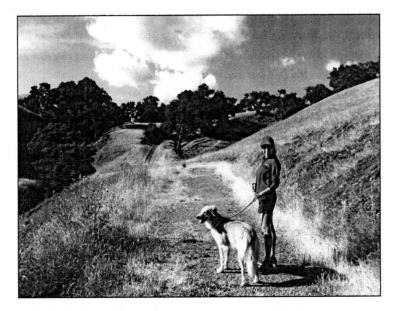

ABOUT THE AUTHOR

Dina Colman, MA, MBA, founded Four Quadrant Living to educate others to live healthier and happier lives by nourishing their Mind, Body, Relationships, and Environment. She emphasizes a balanced approach that can be used by anyone, regardless of age, previous health, or family history.

Dina graduated Phi Beta Kappa and Cum Laude from Pomona College with a BA in Economics. Following graduation, she worked at Price Waterhouse before obtaining her master's degree in business administration from the Kellogg Graduate School of Management at Northwestern University. She then spent over a decade in the high-tech corporate world in a variety of marketing and business strategy positions.

After her sister was diagnosed with Stage 3 breast cancer, Dina was told that she had an 87% chance of getting the disease herself. This motivated Dina to earn a master's degree in holistic health education, learning how to reduce her risk of getting cancer by changing how she lived her life. Fifteen years later, Dina continues to beat the odds and her sister is cancer-free

Dina inspires and informs others through her writing and one-on-one client sessions. She blogs and shares healthy living resources at her www.fourquadrantliving.com website. Her clients and readers are located throughout the United States and around the world.

~

Dina passionately practices the Four Quadrant Living she shares with others. She lives in Danville, California, 30 miles east of San Francisco. To calm her *mind*, she takes time to snuggle with her cat Hollywood and dog Kora. To keep her *body* active, she is a runner and has completed six marathons—including the Boston Marathon. She enjoys a supportive *relationship* with Dave, her husband of 17 years. She spends much of her free time in the natural *environment*, exploring the numerous trails near her home.

Send Dina your questions and comments via email to readers@fourquadrantliving.com.

Please join Four Quadrant Living's online community

on Facebook (FourQuadrantLiving),

on Twitter (@4QuadrantLiving),

and visit www.FourQuadrantLiving.com

CPSIA information can be obtained at www.ICGtesting.com
Printed in the USA
LVOW08s2038270913

354403LV00001B/1/P